Heart to Heart

Advance Praise from Nurses

As a critical care nurse, I've walked many patients and their families through the death experience whether it was sudden and unexpected, or unavoidable and planned. Clare was indispensable at both.

Through her knowledge and example of unshakable faith she has educated, counseled, and consoled not only patients and families but nurses and doctors during some of the most extraordinarily difficult moments in their lives and careers.

She is an expert in spiritual nourishment of the soul, which is easily overlooked in the medical profession but never neglected in her hands.

I hope her words act as a step by guide to inspire others to do as she does because her actions often state loud and clear what a blessing she truly is.

— Alex M., RN

Clare is a blessing! She brings joy and love to the staff and our patients.

— Donna B., RN

A nurse. Overwhelmed, feeling powerless to comfort her patient, to help her peers, to find motivation. Then Clare appears. With her calm, focused, attentive listening she guides me to find my inner wisdom.

I am able to remember in those chaotic moments why I answered the call to nursing and the great purpose I have. Her support and encouragement continue to inspire me in this profession.

Clare's the bomb!

— Mary R., RN

Clare has an instinctive way of focusing on truly what's being said. Her reflective response triggers conversations and stimulates personal thoughts and ideas critical to clinicians in understanding the holistic patient perspectives.

She is a true champion of the bio-psycho-social-SPIRITUAL aspect of nursing care. Blessings and many thanks for bringing the art of listening to our toolbox of care.

— Layne M., RN

Working with Clare was a joyful experience! She exuded warmth, kindness and compassion to every patient, nurse and staff member who were fortunate enough to be in her presence.

— Claudia J., RN

Heart to Heart

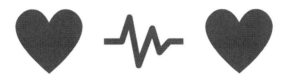

Spiritual Care through Deep Listening

Clare Biedenharn, D.Min., BCC

Printed in the United States of America
First Printing, 2020

ISBN: 978-1-7349242-0-6 (paperback)
ISBN: 978-1-7349242-1-3 (Kindle edition)
Library of Congress Control Number: 2020906953

Published by Page Beyond Press (A Page Beyond LLC)
www.APageBeyond.com

Ordering Information:
Special discounts are available on quantity purchases by corporations, associations, and others who purchase directly from the author. Contact *drclare@yourlisteningpartner.com* for details.

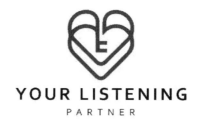

Dedication

There is one reason that we as healthcare providers exist, and that is the patient. The relationship between the patient and those providing care is sacred. I give thanks to all who daily stand as advocates and healers for people at such vulnerable moments of life. Our lives are better because of you.

It is tempting to say that in my work as a critical care chaplain, I served as spiritual director to adrenaline junkies, but that is not quite accurate. The adrenaline edge I witnessed comes not necessarily by choice, but in response to what nurses face in many hospitals: the structure of the hospital itself, including short staffing, twelve-hour shifts, short lunches, and increasing duties that are often technical and complicated. As a chaplain, I met my nurses where they were. That might be in the break room, walking with them between patient rooms, or standing in silent prayer as they entered in response to a Code or Rapid Response call. Providing an additional tool to help them in their jobs was one goal of my study.

Most special to me are the East Jefferson General Hospital (EJGH) nurses that I came to know and love. They welcomed me into their world and fully entered into my learning process. I am a better person for having had the privilege of working beside them each day.

Of course, none of this would have been possible without the support of myriad friends and especially family. My sons, Jay and Robert, grew up with a mother who kept one eye on the ballfield and the other on a book. My family never gave up on me, and they wouldn't let me give up either.

And especially to James. Always and everywhere, this wouldn't have happened without him at my side. You are sorely missed.

Acknowledgments

I truly appreciate the educators whose inherent love for learning and deep desire to mentor have shaped my life and ministry. Dr. Dwight Judy, PhD, guided me through two post-graduate degrees. I thank him for his steadfastness, for his vision in seeing the possibilities for ministry in countless settings, and for his understanding and appreciation of chaplaincy.

Dr. Robert Koch, DNSc, and Maryland Koch, MSN, RN, were unrelenting in their support throughout my listening study and the ensuing rewrites of my dissertation.

East Jefferson General Hospital, in Metairie, Louisiana, maintains a culture of nursing research and provided direct support to this project through education assistance and by welcoming the pursuit of nursing excellence through education. I especially thank:

Dr. Barbara Bihm, D.N.S., R.N., and Bernie Cullen, MSN, RN, of EJGH Research Advisory Board set aside their own point of reference to see value in my project idea. They taught me how to do my very first review of the literature and prepped me for the IRB.

My EJGH onsite committee, Donna Block, R.N., Janet Davis, P.T., M.P.H., Brenda Lege, RN, and Lynn Strain, RN, MSN, CCRN, provided a steady dose of enthusiastic direction as we walked together through my coursework and study design.

Mary Rowe, RN, and my 3rd floor nurses. This project could have sidetracked in a thousand ways without your love and support.

Dr. Thomas G. Nuttli, Sr. MD, Medical Director of EJ's ICU encouraged my curious mind and established a community of learning through daily rounds.

Margaret Janssen, M.S.N, R.N., welcomed this Southern Sojourner into her Northern home for each of my seminary doctoral sessions. She was a nurse and an educator. I am eternally grateful for that day over tea when I said I was packing up and going home. She smiled sweetly and said, "Of course! But I never took you for a quitter!" You won that round, Margaret. I finished, but not before your death. Thanks, my friend.

The EJGH Pastoral Care Department, Rev. Dr. JoAnn Garma, Rev. Lauren Frazier, and Gwen Hammond provided unwavering support as they steered me through the ups and downs of research. They gave me the blessing of a safe place within which to study, ponder, and grow.

Contents

Foreword

by Jean Watson

Clare Biedenharn has offered a gift to nurses and patients alike. Her own study and research on 'Listening' ended up serving as a spiritual awakening and service to self and others. Her Chaplain-based 'Listening Model' was offered as a spiritual practice to nurses, and in turn was transformative to herself. Clare reveals this deep insight and wisdom through her inquiry and inner journey.

The book unfolds not only the 'Listening Model' of authenticity and intentional guides for ways of being. It becomes a living exemplar of transpersonal caring and a caring moment, integrating nursing theory with chaplaincy wisdom teaching and trans-disciplinary caring practices. What is profound in this book is Clare's expert weaving of scripture, ancient knowledge and Biblical sources, and even Nightingale, eliciting evocative, inspiring, and inspirited messages that ground and deepen her teachings.

In addition, Clare Biedenharn offers vignettes of personal active, intentional, authentic 'listening' – with and through inner moments with self; Clare reveals how she was transformed and transfixed in a given moment. By attending to her inner-self-listening, she was blessed with prophetic and insightful guides as she touched the inner life of others, listening to needs behind words.

This work is a blessing to chaplains, nurses, any health professional, and indeed, any human in need of awakening to the mystery and gifts of touching another's life. The combination of Clare's scripture lessons with her personal lessons affirm that when we touch another's life, we also are touched and transformed. This work provides a basic spiritual, intellectual, experiential, and scriptural blueprint for *listening* to our inner lessons that connect us toward healing our shared humanity.

– Jean Watson, PhD, RN, AHN-BC, FAAN, LL (AAN)
  Founder, Watson Caring Science Institute
  www.watsoncaringscience.org
  Distinguished Professor/Dean Emerita, University of Colorado Denver, College of Nursing
  jean@watsoncaringscience.org

Chapter 1:
It All Begins with a Question

Imagine This

It's almost 3:00 a.m. It's been a long shift, and the monitor at the nurses' station confirms what Caroline's been feeling in her gut ever since she received the patient report eight hours ago. Things aren't going well for Mr. Blalock in Room 4. She's been dreading this because it's not the first time she has had him as a patient. These past six months, he's become a "frequent flyer," and she has been part of his care team for most of his admissions. She can anticipate what's coming.

The family acts surprised upon every admission. They either can't or won't see that each time, it isn't a random acute incident, but just one more step in Mr. Blalock's downward trajectory.

"Not tonight, Lord. Not tonight," she tells herself. "If only he would just hold on for a little while longer ...This one's going to be hard to let go." The emotional investment that gradually worked its way into her heart was now settling into her bones as exhaustion.

The call light comes on for Room 4, and she can't help but groan. She knows what is about to happen. The wife planted herself at bedside on day one. Over time, she's opened up to the nurse about her growing concern regarding her husband. Tonight, there's been a shift in both Mr. and Mrs. Blalock. For him it's physical. For her it is something else.

There is a question that Mrs. Blalock is about to ask, and Caroline already knows what it is.

"What would you do if this were *your* family?"

She's heard that question before. She always dreads it, along with the deep conversation that inevitably follows. She can't or won't tell a wife or son or daughter what to do, no matter how much they struggle. It's like their eyes plead for Caroline to solve it for them, but all she can do is try to support them in their pain.

She hates this part of the job. She got into nursing to heal and fix, not to let death take its stand.

She rises stiffly from her chair and slowly turns towards Room 4. As she moves down the hall, she steels herself for what is about to happen.

But just as she reaches the door, something unexpected happens. Nurse Caroline recalls to herself, "This is exactly what the chaplain was talking about. Mrs. Blalock has her answer already. I just have to help her find it. ...Now, how did that go? I remember. It all begins with a question."

Working Together

I am a Board Certified Chaplain (BCC). For my Doctor of Ministry in Spiritual Direction (D.Min.) degree, I conducted a study with critical care nurses at a 420-bed, multi-faith, nonprofit, and four-time Magnet®-designated hospital.

The purpose of this study was to introduce to registered nurses in the critical care settings a spiritually based method of therapeutic Listening Method and to examine their responses to it. The study explored spiritual awareness in nurses and examined whether the model affected the nurses' perceived patient care (Biedenharn, 2014).

All participants were graduates of an accredited basic nursing program and successfully completed the nursing licensure examination. The participants were employed in acute care clinical areas of the hospital and had experience in assisting families in critical care decisions. The twelve participants were 100 percent female and 94 percent Caucasian. Ages ranged from twenty to 59, with the mean age of 49. Years of experience ranged from less than five years to over thirty years of nursing. Based on the self-reported demographics, eight of the twelve (66.6 percent) identified themselves as not having received spirituality training in nursing school. Seven of the twelve (58 percent) identified themselves as having some self-defined personal training in spirituality from books or informal Bible studies.

The results were positive. In the process of the study, I learned a lot about listening and a lot about nurses. We were a committed team. Over time, I came to know and love "my nurses," as we worked side-by-side in the critical care and stepdown settings. Together, we discovered that an open-heart connection can lead to better listening and a transformed life. Not just the nurses were affected. There was a change in me as well, as we worked together on learning a new way to listen. What I've come to know through my work with nurses is that deep listening can lead to deep connection. Connection leads to better care.

And it all begins with a question:

"How did you come to be a nurse?"

Responses vary. Some reasons are practical ones like, "I know I'll always have a job." But there are other responses that often resonate with a certain truth. Those stories usually include a tale about someone in the family who was sick and how, even at a young age, the person learned to provide care. Love shines through these stories. As they are told, there is often a wistful quality that stands in stark contrast to the modern world of healthcare. Those who can take a moment to remember their story, that inner call to helping another, are the ones who seem to be around to tell about it. The others? They don't seem to have the stamina to withstand the years of physical, emotional, and spiritual challenges that are a foundational part of professional nursing practice in our times.

"How did you come to be a nurse?" remains one of my favorite questions to ask nurses. You might be wondering why I care.

My Story

If I could give you information of my life, it would be to show how a woman of very ordinary ability has been led by God in strange and unaccustomed paths to do in His service what He has done in her. And if I could tell you all, you would see how God has done all, and I nothing.

– Florence Nightingale (2019)

Let me tell you my story. I am a female minister in a mainline Protestant church. For many years I served local churches. In that capacity, I came to know many wonderful folks who are faithfully living out their Christian walk. I visited them in the hospital and in their homes, and I stood with them through thick and thin.

Concurrently, I served the community as an industrial chaplain. The title of chaplain usually brings images of military or hospitals. However, some businesses offer chaplain services through their Employee Assistance Program. I was part of a team of chaplains who put on hard hats and steeled toe shoes weekly, to visit job sites. I visited composite floor companies, lumberyards, and a company that provides cranes and large moving equipment like that used to move houses or commercial buildings. My primary company was a shipyard that made oil rigs from scratch and floated them down the Mississippi River to the Gulf Coast for delivery. The only time I worried was when I heard we were getting a chicken company. My fear was that it was a processing plant, so the night before my first visit, I prepared a "Farewell to Chicken" dinner. Thankfully, I only visited the distribution center.

I worked with and came to know the engineers, welders, pipe fitters, and so many others who allowed me to walk with them on their personal journeys. I heard how weekly trips to the casino were going to win them a down payment on a house. Then I heard tales of how much money they lost instead and their angst about paying the bills. I also married and buried their sweet souls over the years. Some of my favorite memories are of speaking with women welders, or of climbing up on the half-finished oil rigs to visit welders as they took a break and ate their supper.

Embracing My Assignment: East Jefferson General Hospital

In 2009, I entered a Clinical Pastoral Education (CPE) training program at East Jefferson General Hospital (EJGH) in Metairie, Louisiana. This posting was to prepare me for board certification through the Association of Professional Chaplains. Over the years as an industrial chaplain, I handled dicey situations like industrial accidents and crisis management. I felt confident that I could manage the workload of post-hurricane Katrina New Orleans. Besides, I had long-time ties to New Orleans. I was there in college, met my husband over a cup of coffee at Camellia Grill (yes, I picked him up), and both our sons were born at Baptist Hospital on Napoleon Avenue.

My first five years at EJGH were filled with gruesome "Katrina survivor stories," like the diabetic lady who lost her legs after living on a tabletop in her flooded home while she waited a week for rescue workers to come. It wasn't just her home that flooded. The waters covered the whole parish, or county, as it is called in other parts of the country. I was hired permanently for the Critical Care Chaplain position. I thought I was doing a solid job as chaplain, but I had limitations that I needed to work through.

The last church I served had not been a good fit for me. The church declared that I couldn't teach, preach, or lead because I was a woman. I knew that I had been called to

17

ministry, but I wasn't called to take abuse. It had been a rough year. As I climbed out of the wrestling ring, I was more than a little unclear about what I had to offer anyone. In fact, I felt my reserves had been stripped by that assignment. When I arrived for the CPE chaplain residency, I wasn't sure if I had anything left to give.

At the beginning of the program, it was time for unit assignments. The choices whizzed by me. I said a little prayer for guidance. All the assignments were accounted for, except the Intensive Care Unit (ICU) and "stepdown unit," where patients transition from critical care to standard care. Those 58 beds (29 in each unit) seemed like just another version of what I had been doing in an industrial setting. I asked for God's help and trusted God to open the door to where I needed to be. Somehow, this was it.

Like the ICU patients, I came to the third floor of EJGH broken and exhausted. And like many of them, I was healed and restored. I give credit to God and to my nurses for my seven-year journey toward recovery. They took me in, brushed me off, and helped me find the good things about myself. They challenged me, and they loved me. Together we enjoyed a special kind of relationship based on mutual admiration, learning, and ultimately, love. Through them, I rediscovered my own call to service. And to my amazement, so did they.

One More Goal: Doctor of Ministry in Spiritual Direction

I loved my job. I loved my city. I had one more goal: to earn my Doctor of Ministry (D.Min.) in Spiritual Direction. It had been a longtime dream. When I came to the hospital, I quickly learned that the letters trailing behind one's name could be useful. And since I'm an inveterate lifelong learner, it became a possibility. My supervisor supported the goal, as long as the directors of my units would agree to it. I nervously approached the ICU director with my well-practiced sales pitch. When I hesitantly laid out this opportunity to grow in my profession, her response was, "Why would you not?"

The Study

In 2013, I gathered a small group of EJGH critical care and step-down nurses to test whether an ancient listening model could increase spiritual awareness in nurses and affect the nurses' perceived patient care.

The project was anchored in a very common problem.

The Case of Uncle C.H.

As I wrestled with ideas for studies with practical outcomes, the image of Clarence Hungerford ("C.H.") Mackey came to mind. C.H. was my husband's uncle, but from the time I first met him, I claimed him as my own. He was a kind and loving man who was a retired U.S. Army colonel and WWII veteran. I never knew Uncle C.H. to say an unkind word to anyone. He was generous in love and spirit.

Many years earlier, Uncle C.H. had been stricken with Parkinson's disease, as had his brother before him. Having watched his brother's health decline from the disease, Uncle C.H. and Aunt Frances knew what they were up against when his own diagnosis came. Aunt Frances cared for him devotedly for several years, and eventually, the question of placing the feeding tube came up. Uncle C.H. was no longer able to participate in the discussion. As Frances wrestled with the decision, she looked for support in her family, friends, and church.

The day after the feeding tube procedure was performed, my uncle's doctor, who had been a part of the discussion at every step, told Aunt Frances, "I usually don't agree with this decision."

For the next seven years, Uncle C.H. lay at home in a bed, faithfully attended by his wife and with full home health support. He was neither here nor there. He was stuck in a rigid body, unable to respond. More than once, Aunt Frances declared in anguish, "Why didn't that doctor say something *before* the feeding tube operation?"

In all fairness, maybe the doctor had. We all know that patients and loved ones often do what the rest of us do. They hear either what they expect, or what they want to hear, while the rest of the information evaporates or rides off into the sunset.

Activist Parker Palmer: The Disconnect and Rediscovery

Over the years of my coursework, the educator, theorist, and community activist Parker Palmer appeared in various contexts. Required reading for Adult Learning course, *The Courage to Teach* (Palmer, 2007) illuminated the disconnection from what is important in the work that we do. The book reflected a shift from professor-centered learning to student-centered. At the time, I was serving a church while attending school. It struck me that the title of Palmer's 2007 work could easily have been *The Courage to PREACH*.

Reflecting on the deep emotions that book stirred in me, I now see an even broader call. This disconnection can be found in many different professions, including those in healthcare. When what we live out in our daily life resonates with who we are in our hearts, then, as Palmer describes it, we are living an "undivided life" (2013, p. 10). Living the undivided life strengthens us personally. And as our true selves shine, the world reflects back to us our brightness, and we are all strengthened.

Palmer's "undivided life" (2013, p. 10) models for us the possibilities. He first came to this realization through his work as an educator. Over time, his body of work expanded to include leadership in a variety of settings, including healthcare and business.

Palmer continued to show up on my assigned reading lists. In seminary we read several of his books and articles. A common thread throughout Palmer's work is rediscovering the heart's call to one's chosen work, while making the world a better place.

Palmer draws heavily on the inclusive Quaker faith traditions of service and peace. The more I read, the more I was inspired to rediscover how my life – both personally and professionally – reflected my lifelong call to serve.

The Model

My "Aha!" moment came in seminary as I read a book about Quaker practices. I saw a term that was like coming home for me: "Theology of the Heart" (Graham et al, 2005). I thought to myself, "*That's* why I do what I do..."

I continued to read and discovered that the Quakers, also known as the Society of Friends, believe that God is within each of us, and that by waiting and being open to the possibility, God's Wisdom may make itself known. Expectant waiting and listening are the basis for their worship, their community life, and their personal decision making. When someone is wrestling with a question like whether to change jobs or whom to marry, they can request that a few people sit with them to ask questions about the matter at hand. This is called a "Clearness Committee," because its focus is on clearing up confusion about the important questions in life. Using open questions can often help draw out the wisdom from within to help the individual make a decision.

Basic Quaker tenets of inclusiveness ("FAQs", 2018) make it an especially helpful model of spiritual care in the hospital setting, as they include a belief that God is within each of us. This in turn anchors their approach to living, as evidenced by their embrace of the multi-cultural, multi-racial stance and their historical commitment to social justice ("The Social Justice Testimony | Quaker Information Center", 2020).

The more I read and the more I observed the full range of situations at the hospital, the idea bubbled up that intentional use of this reflective listening model could be employed at the bedside. Perhaps by adapting the Quakers' "Clearness Committee" model, nurses could help people like Uncle C.H. and Aunt Frances face the tough questions. Perhaps a nurse could help patients tap into the wisdom that lies within, so that patients could find their own answers.

Study Site

As part of the requirements for my degree, I taught this listening model to a small group of nurses. The study of nurses affirmed that intentional listening affected both the nurses and patient care.

The study site was East Jefferson General Hospital (EJGH), the first Louisiana hospital to receive the coveted Magnet® designation, and the only one to receive it four times. Nursing research continues to be an important part of EJGH culture. At the suggestion of my onsite committee, I approached the Nurse Research Department to participate in the review of the literature as well as the study design. Under their direction, the study proposal passed the challenging hospital Institutional Review Board (IRB). My seminary's Human Subjects Committee approved the study the same week. The way was now clear.

Study Design

Design of the study evolved over a period of two years, beginning with discussion with the members of the onsite committee. Of the five members of the committee, three were seasoned registered nurses (RNs), each with over thirty years of nursing experience. The remaining members were both deacons in their respective denominations as well as EJGH hospital administrators. The committee included the directors of the two critical care units involved in the study and the Director of Pastoral Care.

The final number of participants was small. Sixteen RNs originally volunteered to participate in the study, but the final number was twelve, due to scheduling conflicts. Each participant:

- Graduated from an accredited nursing program
- Successfully completed the nursing licensure examination
- Was currently licensed as a registered nurse (RN)
- Was employed full-time in acute care clinical areas of EJGH
- Had experience in assisting families in critical care decisions

The participants were 100 percent female, 94 percent Caucasian, and 6 percent African American. Ages ranged from a 20- to 29-year range to a 50- to 59-year range, with a mean age of 49. Years of experience ranged from under five to over thirty years of nursing practice.

Based on the self-reported demographics, eight of the twelve (66.6 percent) identified as not having received spirituality training in nursing school. Seven of the twelve (58 percent) identified as having some type of self-defined personal training in spirituality, such as through books or informal Bible studies.

Five Steps of the Study

There were five steps to the study:

1. Participants completed a demographic survey followed by a pre-Daily Spiritual Experience Scale (DSES) survey to measure basic daily spirituality (Underwood, 2003). The DSES Scale was initially designed as a measurement of spirituality for research in the healthcare setting and has been used in studies worldwide.

2. Participants viewed a PowerPoint presentation featuring the Quaker Listening Model, followed by discussion.

3. The researcher conducted a series of three semi-structured interviews with each participant, intended to occur every two weeks. These one-on-one discussions were based on open questions concerning the use of the model as an effective listening tool.

4. Participants completed a post DSES survey.

5. The researcher conducted an in-depth taped interview with eight participants who volunteered to participate by indicating on the post DSES survey their willingness to do so.

I taught the Quaker Listening Model (based on the Clearness Committee concept, described in detail in Chapter 9) and followed up with three interviews two weeks apart. In addition, half the participants agreed to taped interviews. They all signed informed consent forms that allowed for use of the interviews with the condition that the participants remain anonymous.

This is my story. It is shaped by the people who walked with me as I have walked with others. My D.Min. project was a collaborative effort. My background is in theology, so learning the clinical walk was part of my steep learning curve. Critical care nurses helped me formulate my project, even as I was teaching them the centuries-old Quaker Listening Method. Over the course of the study, I interviewed them and listened to their responses to a simple and effective type of listening. I dedicate this book to those nurses, to my family, and to all the nurses who can't imagine doing anything else. Their love of nursing makes our world better.

My nurses taught me this valuable work was easy to apply and had a positive effect on their patient care, as they remembered the compassionate "why?" behind my question.

So, tell me, how did you come to be a nurse?

Points to Ponder

I answered the call to ministry and started seminary in my 40s. I received my master's degree in Spiritual Formation and an Education Specialist (Ed.S.) degree in Adult Learning in my 50s. I was in my 60s when I finally received my Doctoral degree.

Do You Have a Dream?

- Do you have a personal or professional "itch" you need to scratch?
- What's keeping you from achieving it or even starting towards it?
- What are you afraid of?
- When you self-identify as a nurse, can you name your strongest emotion?
- What's your least favorite part?
- For you, what is the best part of being a nurse?

...And You Might Try

Take some time to remember your own story. How did you come to be a nurse?

Keeping track of our feelings can be challenging at the best of times. Journaling can be a way to capture and name those feelings. A journal can also provide the opportunity to reflect upon your feelings. Could you share your nursing story in a journal or with a colleague or a friend?

Reading this book might bring up feelings within you, and feelings about your profession may surface. A journal can be an effective tool for tracking your feelings and reflecting on your responses.

As you look back on your call to nursing, what would you tell that younger, less experienced version of yourself as he/she began on the very first day of the very first job? Consider writing your younger self a letter about that new life in nursing.

Chapter 2:
The Bottom Line

God spoke to me and called me to His Service. What form this service was to take the voice did not say.

– Florence Nightingale
(Bostridge, 2008)

The Basis: To Be in Service

Sure we had our breakdown and felt hopeless. And then our jobs and why we do what we do came back to reality. We need to save our patients and ourselves. If we were going to die today, we would at least do it protecting others and do everything we can to live... And we did! We were an awesome team of mostly strangers doing whatever we could and had to do – and we did phenomenally! (Johnson, 2018)

– Tamara Ferguson RN

These are the words of a labor and delivery nurse who was part of the healthcare team responsible for evacuating patients from the burning Adventist Feather Hospital in the infamous November 2018 Paradise, California, wildfire. As flames threatened the hospital, the staff evacuated patients who represented a full array of acuity from fresh cesarean birth to critically ill. Ferguson and another nurse were responsible for a group who, after they left the hospital, remained trapped in the flames. They sequestered the patients in a nearby garage, the only safe space they could find. They stretched the patients out on the concrete floor and kept them as comfortable as possible. Through texts and phone calls, they were discovered, eventually rescued, and brought to safety.

This is the quality of nurse that I know. I cannot think of a single nurse who would not have done the same thing.

Recently, I reconnected with some of the nurses who participated in the study. Over lunch I shared with them what has since become my personal mission: "To help healthcare workers reconnect to their call to service. Deep listening leads to deep connection." Those words drew strong response from the full range of my nurses, from professional substance abuse counselors that I addressed at a community college, and from a physical therapist struggling with burnout. In each environment, the unanimous response was, "YES! We need this!"

May I Be of Help?

How may I be of service to you? How can I help you to rediscover the motivation to provide consistent, professional care? Care that meets the standards of professional nursing, as well as meeting the institutional standards of your employer? More importantly, I refer to the care that you don't brag about, because it is simply a part of who you are. It is a matter of personal integrity.

Sometimes it is difficult to remain true to that quality while following today's business model of hospital care. The nurse is tasked with a higher ratio of high acuity patients, while managing complicated technical procedures, as well as carrying out the necessary charting. Every day is challenging. What can you do for yourself to avoid burnout, fatigue, frustration, and sometimes even a sense of hopelessness?

If there is a magic 1-2-3 formula, it has not presented itself yet. However, you are not without tools. Within you there is strength, persistence, and love. My goal is to help you remember and rediscover the resources that you have but may have dismissed or even forgotten.

What "feeds" you in your profession? What is it about your work, aside from paying the bills, that calls to you each day?

As one of my study nurses described it:

"...When you slow down you feel closer to God. And you do realize why you are here. And it's not necessarily the paycheck, even though I say that it is. It's not. So it's really what your whole purpose in life is. To be able to serve. For me, it's to do a good job while I'm here, but also to make a difference in people" (Participant #12).

The call to be a part of something bigger than ourselves, to make a difference, can sustain us through the toughest times.

My Story... Again

I ask these questions because I had to ask them of myself as I reconnected with my own call to service. The study focused on my nurses, but I also became more self-aware during this process. I had come to the hospital feeling broken. Through the work with the listening project, I once again caught a whiff of what drove my work in ministry for over twenty years. I thought finishing the project was the pinnacle of my professional life, but I had missed something.

A doctorate was my dream, and the opportunity to work on it in a hospital was like icing on the cake. The course work was finished. The project was designed and approved. My nurses and I completed the study, and I was winding up the dissertation in the fall of 2013. I combed the study results and gleaned the themes that anchored the work. It was a concrete, wonderful time.

Walking the Fence

In March 2014, I headed from New Orleans to Chicago to defend my dissertation at my seminary. My doctoral work was not accepted by my committee. I was turned down and told to head back to the drawing board. If my goal had simply been getting a few additional letters behind my name, that would have been one thing. This was something else. What began as a seemingly simple project now compelled me to follow through to the finish. I owed it to my nurses who gave me their time, energy, and support. I also felt that my efforts were contributing to the Greater Good. This was my call to service.

The main problem with the project was that I was delicately walking the fence between the worlds of nursing/healthcare and theology. Historically, the two were linked. In the earliest days, Greek temples had formalized treatments for illnesses and designated places of healing. Hospitals as we now know them evolved from medieval monasteries that were hospices, providing care for religious pilgrims. In those days, what little passed for medical care belonged to the rich. Care consisted primarily of attempts to support the body in healing itself, as there was little to offer compared to today.

In general, the broad brush of medicine and spirituality share a long history based on compassionate care. Florence Nightingale's call to serve expressed itself through radical transformation of the existing patient care model of her time. Barbara Dossey, a nurse and Nightingale scholar, highlighted in a lecture (2001) at the Washington National Cathedral that service was anchored in a deep connection to God. However, in the Western empirical medical model, the importance of spirituality is minimized. This is changing.

Changing Models

There is a resurgence of interest in the holistic health model as the medical/healthcare community seeks to respond to patient expectations based on an increased interest in spirituality as well as increased access to information from the Internet. The response to the consumer demands reignites discussion between the disciplines of science and spirituality, even as it butts up against the insurance companies who dictate modes of healthcare delivery.

The holistic health care model is based on reconnecting with the ancient understanding of the multifaceted nature of the patient (Valizadeh et al., 2017). The concept is that the whole patient's spiritual, mental, and physical natures are integrated and expressed as parts of a single unit. Spiritual assessment is an essential element of this understanding. True to form, data is the key to current assessment because it can be easily entered into the electronic chart. Information gleaned in the assessment determines patient care.

The Joint Commission (JCAHO), the national accrediting agency responsible for accreditation guidelines for all areas of the hospital, requires spiritual assessment (Lewis, 2008). However, JCAHO does not explicitly assign that responsibility to any specific member of the interdisciplinary healthcare team. Nurses, social workers, or chaplains can perform the assessment, although the gatekeeper is often the bedside nurse. Yet myriad studies show that spiritual care is not an area that many nurses are comfortable with, either professionally or personally (Jenkins, 2009).

A nurse in the emergency department once said to me, "Go in and do what you do. I don't understand it, but you always make people feel better." It often works that way for patients as well as for staff.

"It's like serving a church as a minister. The staff are your Sunday regulars and the patients are the visitors. The patients come and go, but you build long relationships with the staff," a wise hospital chaplain once told me.

The hospital chaplain role is in transition. Hospitals are shifting away from the strong historical ties to spiritual-based hospitals. In the process, a mixture of attitudes is emerging, both by and toward chaplains. As hospitals operate more in a business-based model, chaplains are scrambling to establish themselves not only as persons of God but also as recognized healthcare professionals. Maintaining board certification through the Association of Professional Chaplains requires fifty hours of continuing education per year, including five hours of research. Apparently, we professional chaplains are working hard to prove ourselves *to ourselves,* as well as to the healthcare community.

To be a chaplain is to be an outlier, and this has its inherent challenges as one who remains detached from the main body. Although I am endorsed by the church, my ministry setting is beyond its physical walls. Some clergy and seminary professors don't understand it to be valid ministry. When I told one professor that I might be the only religious authority a patient might know, I was dismissed as being arrogant. On the other hand, in the culture of today, minimizing my church connection may allow me to minister to someone who doesn't claim a particular church or who may have bad feelings towards organized religion.

Long, long ago an old man and his wife decided that God wasn't fulfilling a promise made to them in the way they expected, so they took it upon themselves to make things happen by having a child by the maidservant. Finally, God came to that couple, Sarah and Abraham, and gave them a child who would be a part of a greater plan to sustain God's people for all time. However, God also came to Hagar, Sarah's abandoned maid, and Ishmael, son of Abraham, and created for them a separate, valid plan. A chaplain comes to everyone, no matter what their faith, and helps each person find the spiritual resources within.

My belief is that God has a way of shaping our circumstances as God wants them to be. We are not alone as we face whatever life or work throws at us. Our call to service is a call to be a part of something bigger than we are. And as we do this, we have an opportunity to grow in every facet of our lives.

With clarifying help and support from two incredible nurse educators, my work was completed and approved. I graduated in 2015 with a Doctor of Ministry in Spiritual Direction (D.Min.) from Garrett Theological Seminary in Evanston, Illinois.

Remembering the Connection

One of my study nurses told me about her experience in church as she listened to the words of the sermon encouraging all to be sensitive to the needs of others.

"I thought, 'This is what I do as a nurse.' And I thought about how closely what we do aligns with God's plan to treat others as we would like to be treated. And I thought about what we do is a journey, and that I'm not going to be deterred." And she repeated, "I am *not* going to be deterred" (Participant #5).

She caught the connection between being kind to others and the meaning of her work. At that moment, she recommitted herself to service.

The challenge lies in remembering this call in a world that focuses on individuality in every aspect of life, including our relationship with God. Florence Nightingale, the founder of modern nursing, lived within a culturally supported Christianity, but we do not. She had an established daily spiritual practice including prayer and meditation, but many of us do not.

Just as she fought to establish a new level of care, today's nurses struggle to maintain those standards in the face of a business/finance model which may no longer be faith-based. For those whose heart lies in patient care and safety, the odds of consistently providing a high level of care is sometimes daunting. Yet for those who are truly called to this work, this is the essence of their being. You may be performing nursing tasks, but a nurse is who you are.

This was vividly illustrated to me one cold day. There was a small fire in the nursing home immediately behind the hospital. Their safety plan included evacuating nursing home residents to the halls of the hospital. All available hospital staff were called to provide support, as patients were rolled in from across the street. As the halls filled, I watched the hospital's Chief Nursing Officer and the Director of Care Management, both RNs, instinctively step back into the bedside nursing role, central to their being, as they moved among the patients, directing care.

Knowledge, critical thinking, skill, and most importantly compassion are core elements of the work you do.

So how may I be of service to you?

Points to Ponder

- What does service mean to you?
- If you had to give up everything but one thing about your job, what would that one thing be?
- Do you have a place to stash your worries?
- In what way does life intrude and distract you?
- In what way might busyness be a buffer to prevent authentic engagement with your patients, your coworkers, or your family?

...And You Might Try

As you well know, breath is essential to life. As you go through your day, try noticing your breath. If we're anxious, the breath is often shallow. Stop. Take as deep a breath as you are comfortable with (at least at the beginning). Let it out slowly.

Remember the old saying about doing artificial resuscitation: In with the good air, out with the bad.

Once you notice your breath, you might take it a step further:

- Before you enter the patient's room, stop and take a breath.
- Breathe in on the count of four. Hold for the count of seven.
- Release and count to eight.
- You are clearing out your old energy, burdens, or just plain junk before you enter the room to meet your next patient. You are creating an opening, a clear playing field.

Chapter 3:
Spiritual Care as Practice

How very little can be done under the spirit of fear. I am of certain convinced that the greatest heroes are those who do their duty in the daily grind of domestic affairs whilst the world whirls as a maddening dreidel.

– Florence Nightingale (2019)

"I am an emotional person. When I began nursing I had to find the boundary between my emotions and my professional distance. I think I found it out now I'm looking at it more. This [listening] method has me thinking about it in a different way" (Participant #14).

Let's pretend for a minute that you are preceptor to a recent nursing school graduate. How would you respond to the question, "What IS spiritual care?" Write down your answer.

If you can't reel off a standard response to what constitutes spiritual care in ten words or less, don't feel bad.

Understanding spiritual care is challenging because it is so broad and yet so personal for both you and your patient.

Repeatedly, throughout the literature, spiritual care is a puzzle. A very big elephant in a very small room. It's broad and wide and something people talk around, but have trouble describing. Yet spiritual care is a familiar phrase in the nursing lexicon. The Joint Commission (JCAHO) requires a spiritual assessment, which often falls to nurses who may have little or no formal training in the process. Even though we want a list we can check off and proudly mark 'Done,' spiritual care stubbornly remains outside of the wrap-it-up-and-stick-it-in-a-box comfort that we seek. Describing spiritual care in the hospital setting is challenging within the healthcare vocabulary.

- **Quantifiable:** Is there an insurance code for providing spiritual care? Physicians can be reimbursed for a palliative consult, but general spiritual care appears more elusive. If there were, what would be the measurement? What numbers could be used? How do you quantify the outcome of something like attentive listening?
- **Specific:** A longing to be a part of something bigger than our personality is a universal response. Not everyone is religious, but spirituality lies in the "we" of the collective mind. What brings spiritual comfort to one does not necessarily translate to spiritual comfort for another.
- **Impersonal:** Where does God come into your life? Many nurses have not considered in what way their own beliefs and

history affect what they hear and how they respond. Personal experience shapes our expectations. We hear what we expect to hear, which is personal.

Finding the Niche

Religion and spirituality are established as two distinct ideas within the current literature. *Religion* is described as a corporate faith community that shares a prescribed set of beliefs. *Spirituality*, on the other hand, refers to seeking the presence of God around you. While spirituality is often the focus in the healthcare setting, don't underestimate the power of religion in one's life. It can be a great source of comfort for individuals who depend on their religion to find meaning.

What might all disciplines agree upon as basic spiritual care? To begin with, spirituality includes the essential question of what makes us human. This would include respect for the individual, respect for privacy, and other cultural and religious needs.

The Rugged Individualist remains a strong model in the world thanks to John Wayne, Rambo, and any number of sci-fi movies. In this climate, the question of how the importance of religion is linked to spirituality may be overlooked. A person who has never been to church or does not practice a spiritual regimen may not fully understand how important those facets of life might be for a patient, the family, or even co-workers. The format of religion can be a powerful source of individual and corporate strength, which is why awareness of cultural diversity is important to providing spiritual care.

For example, spiritual care means different things to different people. Imagine a patient is sitting in the middle of the room. If the patient represents a whole person requiring holistic healthcare, each professional person making an assessment within individual disciplines could represent facets that combine to make the whole person. Each assessment is based on a specific set of criteria established by the profession represented. The intent may be a clear, non-biased assessment, but human nature creeps in. The chaplain or minister sees assessment from one perspective. Social workers, care managers, and those representing the medical model may have other perspectives. In addition, each of those assessments is affected by both personal and professional bias. Most likely, the truth lies in a composite of the assessments.

One time I was called to the ICU to support a dying Jewish patient and her family prior to one of the High Holy Days. The tenets they followed were more conservative than other Jewish individuals I had worked with before. When the rabbi arrived, I spoke with him and touched his shoulder. The patient's husband looked alarmed and said, "You might need to talk to somebody about that." I was confused until our chaplain resident, who was herself a rabbi, whispered to me that I could not touch him. I was a woman. Immediately I got the connection. The rabbi had probably gone through ritual cleansing before the holiday, so being touched by a female would be considered unacceptable within his culture.

Cultural awareness in spiritual care is important. I have a confession. As a postmenopausal woman, I just don't think about that stuff anymore. In my faith, ritual cleansing is not practiced, so it is not on my consideration radar. However, this wasn't about me. I was at fault for not being more culturally aware. My reaction was not to take it personally or to put it in my world. My concern was that my unknowing goof might interfere with the patient and her family receiving the ritual support that they craved and that only their rabbi could provide.

Don't Force It

An old saying talks about how trying to put a square peg in a round hole is difficult. Two rigid edges not meant to fit together clash. In a way, that is what different religions can do. If we come with a set of beliefs and try to mold the spiritual care of the patient to our own philosophies, we are doing an injustice to the patient and to ourselves.

A skill that chaplains are known for is called "reading the room." When a chaplain first comes into a situation, it is important to pause, listen, and discern what is going on, who the players are, and what the need might be. The chaplain responds to the perceived need and shapes the response to address that specific need. The chaplain's aim is to meet the needs of those present, not impose the chaplain's needs.

I was placed in an awkward position when I recorded an interview with one of my study nurses, a devoted Christian. The struggle for me was to remain the neutral interviewer as she explained how she shared Christ with a patient discharged home on hospice. It did not go well:

"He was ready to die but he hadn't addressed his faith or anything. Nothing like that. I was able to share with him, but it was discouraging because he was just like, 'Well, that's fine.' But as a believer I couldn't let it go. It's like 'No, you need to address this! This is not worth giving up on.' It was just discouraging because I know this guy is going home to die. And to be not adamant but nonchalant like 'That's fine if Jesus is for you' ...This is not something to just casually blow off" (Participant #5).

Like forcing a square peg into a round hole, the conversation was not about the patient but about the nurse's missional need to share her faith. Her intentions were good from her perspective, but ultimately the conversation was about her need, not the patient's.

Her specific desires and his general needs were not in sync. She held the power in that relationship, and she misread the situation. She was hearing his responses, but not listening to what he was trying to convey. What she heard wasn't satisfying her own needs, so she kept talking, not listening. Because she brought a personal agenda, she missed an opportunity to be present for her patient. She missed a rare moment, found in the gift of full engagement. Quickly it can slip away.

Spiritual care is delicate work. The temptation is to simply request a pastoral care consult. There are no right answers in providing spiritual care, except those that bring comfort and help the individual find meaning.

Sometimes when people hear of my chaplain experience, they say, "Wow. I bet that's a great place to bring people to Jesus." My answer is, "No." My role may represent a Higher Power to those who are vulnerable, but the work is not about evangelism. My call is to provide compassionate care and help individuals tap into the resources they already have within.

Spiritual Care Is About You, Too

For some nurses, providing spiritual care is merely one of the tasks that they perform. Maybe they love it, and maybe they don't. It is still a solid place to be. For others, it represents something else. As I scored the pre- and post- tests of the Daily Spiritual Experience Scale (Underwood, 2003) for the study, I noted beginning test results were quite high. I mentioned that to one of the study nurses and her response was:

"Our job...We have such a wonderful spot to be such a blessing for so many people...It's very spiritual. I see my job as being in a unique spot for people...You know you see them on the street, maybe they're not very, well...They could even be scary...but then I think, "Wow. You could be in my hospital bed and I would be holding your hand petting you." And she laughs, "I wouldn't be afraid. But they are so vulnerable then so you're in such a unique spot to minister to those people when you couldn't on the street or walking around town. So I find nursing so spiritual" (Participant #13).

I worked with a nurse who cared for a patient with internal decapitation. The patient appeared intact, but the spine was separated from the skull. The patient had been injured in a motor vehicle accident, and – against the odds – she woke up. Although paralyzed and ventilator dependent, she was able to respond to yes or no questions by blinking her eyes. The nurse opened up to me about his lack of belief in a formal religion. He stated that he did not believe in God; he saw this accident as a result of the Law of Probability. To him, this was basically an example of being in the wrong place (or the wrong car) at the wrong time.

However, less than an hour earlier, the prayer team at the patient's church heard that she was beginning to respond. They brought her a prayer shawl, laid hands on her, and prayed for healing. It may appear that there would be no middle ground of connection between the beliefs of the patient and those of the nurse, but that is what makes bedside care special. The nurse was able to support the patient's needs without judgment. Awareness, training, and desire assist in finding that sweet spot.

The Hang-ups

One could say that healthcare providers sometimes view the world differently from theologians. The practices of medicine and nursing are ideally based upon best practices that are examined and confirmed by quantifiable research. Conversely, theology and the humanities generally deal with unquantifiable themes such as faith and hope. Tension between these disciplines may be linked to the lack of common ground and common language. Yet this relationship is evolving with an increased emphasis on spiritual care.

Historically, care for others has come from a base of compassion. The current high-efficiency model of healthcare encourages spirituality to be placed in a medical-model box that can be checked off as completed. What are the implications of reducing spiritual care to a set of acronyms that can be printed on a pocket card? Seeking a quick fix causes us to miss the invitation to go a little deeper.

In all fairness, the nature of spiritual care is complicated. How do you grab it? Its diversity makes it hard to define or understand, let alone carry it out with integrity. There is no gold standard, and there shouldn't be. Providing spiritual care is shaped by individual interaction, one patient at a time. Maybe *that* is the gold standard.

The literature indicates that most nurses feel unprepared to fully engage in the spiritual assessment and care of patients. In 2010, the United Kingdom Royal College of Nursing commissioned an online survey of the nurse experience of spiritual care. The results indicated 83.4 percent felt that providing spiritual care was fundamental to nursing care, while 79.3 percent felt that lack of education remains a major block obstacle to providing that specialized care. As one respondent stated in the Royal College final survey:

"If medicine involves the recovery of the body, then spiritual care...involves a recovery of the patient as a person. These areas do not sit in contention, but aim to complement each other and serve to remind us that 'there is no profit in curing the body if in the process we destroy the soul'" (Respondent Nurse) ("RCN Spirituality Survey 2010", 2011).

One of the difficulties in providing spiritual care to patients is that there is no single quantifiable, specific spiritual experience. Any definition of spiritual care is ambiguous and will always be so, by its very nature. This ambiguity leads to subjectivity and to personal interpretation.

This is anathema to the modern medical model, which is more skills-based. Studies show that nurses want to know what personal spiritual care is, so that they may provide it within the boundaries of personal belief and professional practice.

Within the holistic healthcare model concept in many nursing theory models, the patient's spiritual, mental, and physical natures are considered integrated. Nurses are encouraged to assess the patient's spiritual needs and include the assessment in the plan of care.

However, practice does not always successfully transfer from theory. The lack of discussion may be a detractor from fully embracing holistic spiritual care. Reasons for avoiding the discussion can be as simple as:

- We're too busy.
- We don't have time or the right words.
- We don't know what spirituality is.

Spiritual Care 101: The Basics

The importance of spiritual care is not new to clinicians, but the process can seem abstract and awkward at first. These acronyms can be very effective tools to guide the assessment. FICA and HOPE are two of the better-known mnemonics. They are taught in many disciplines and considered to be effective in guiding the assessment.

FICA

Faith and Belief: What is the thread one holds onto as a coping mechanism in stressful situations?

Importance: How does this belief shape who you are as a person? How important is it to you?

Community: Are there others around you who share your beliefs? Do you have a faith community for support?

Address in Care: What does the care team need to do address any concerns the patient may have? (Puchalski & Ferrell, 2010)

HOPE

Hope: Where does your hope lie?

Organized Religion: Are you a part of a faith community? If you are, is it meaningful to you?

Personal Spirituality / Practice: Are there practices you are committed to? Are they meaningful to you?

Effects: How does your belief affect your needs? How does it affect end-of-life choices? (Anandarajah & Hight, 2001)

These are helpful tools. There is another step, however: application. The same set of acronyms can yield different results based on how they are applied. Assessment can be done *to* a patient, but it can also be done *with* the patient. Each approach can yield different results.

Imagine this scenario.

Sally, a 14-year-old-girl, watches a tennis match on TV, and she is inspired to try the sport. She goes to the attic and grabs an old racket and some balls she found up there. She watches a few YouTube videos and now feels she can master the game. Her first step is hitting the ball against the garage door. It's fun, and as she practices, she gains confidence.

One day, she finds out her school friend Shasta is doing the same thing. She has an old racket. She watched the YouTube videos. She also enjoys hitting tennis balls, and her garage door is as battered as Sally's. They decide to meet at the tennis court to hit a few balls back and forth. Each has been trying it solo. Now they want to see what it is like to volley the ball between two people. That makes the game very different. Hitting the ball against the garage was somewhat static. The garage has no emotional commitment. Hitting the ball between two people is dynamic.

Imagine spiritual assessment tools as a structure that assists in making a connection. The practitioner guides the assessment, just like the tennis rules guide the girls' game. The tools keep the conversation focused and on track.

In Sally and Shasta's game, both need to understand the framework, and both have to play to make it work. Each girl brings her own set of skills and expectations to the game. The connection between them is what is important about the game, and the results are often unexpected.

Many assessment tools focus primarily on the patient. The moments at bedside, when the nurse and the patient each bring something to the exchange, can provide a different kind of connection. Jean Watson calls it "the caring moment" where two people are authentically present and engaged (Bevis & Watson, 2000). That moment includes being present, connected, and intentional, just like the girls on the tennis court.

The spiritual assessment tools are important parts of your toolbox. Everything else is enhancement.

Religion

Aside from what your personal beliefs might be, don't underestimate how important a patient's religion may be in providing comfort, relief, and order. Religion offers structure. There is a standard set of beliefs for that particular faith. Common language helps explain experience. A sense of belonging can bring profound peace and comfort.

- Try to set your personal beliefs and biases aside, so that you can provide support for your patients' religious beliefs and expressions without prejudice.
- Acknowledge religion's importance to patients.
- Support any religious practices patients may have.
- Allow easy access to their religious leaders.
- Call the chaplain to support both the patient and you.

Nonreligious

Spiritual-but-not-religious is a broad designation that covers everything other than formal religion. What is spiritual to you may not be spiritual to the next person, but that doesn't invalidate its importance to either of you. Deep connection is a longing of humanity, and its impulse draws us to a spiritual journey.

Some find their spiritual place in nature or in private prayer. Some of us pray without ceasing, as the Apostle Paul instructs. If that's the case, any thought that is directed to a Higher Power could be considered a prayer. I pray for parking spaces. I pray for our world and for the staff and families who are in my care. My practices are shaped by my personal religious upbringing and training, but they are not dependent on formal church. I find this to be true for many people, especially for those who have been disappointed by a church experience.

The desire for a connection with a higher force continues. In many faiths, light is used as image of God. "The human spirit is the lamp of the Lord that sheds light on one's inmost being" (Proverbs 20:27, New International Version). Buddhists, Jewish mystics, *The Koran*, and Christianity all include the image of light in the search for the divine.

In this confusing setting of trying to capture a definition of spiritual care, what specific actions can you take? Here are some places to start.

Make Eye Contact

Eyes are said to be gateways to the soul. Making contact with your eyes is affirming. It's like you are saying, "You are real. I am real. We've got this."

Use Their Name

We depersonalize without thinking sometimes. The "gallbladder in 426" or the "stroke in 13" is a convenient form of identification. But it is also a way to distance and protect ourselves from interaction.

Ask patients what name they prefer. This can bring all kinds of responses. Some cultures use a lot of nicknames. I go by my middle name, Clare. When I hear my first name, Dorothy, I either don't recognize it as me or my guard goes up, because usually it's associated with something official. One of my doctors has a note in my record so they can consistently address me as Clare, the name I prefer to use. It may seem like a small gesture, but I appreciate their effort.

> *"A room number and the room number's condition is very disassociating from being an actual person. So we take the time to listen to their needs and then you kind of connect with them and it's not just a room number any more or a disease or whatever...And so I think you see more of a person instead of just a patient." (Participant #5)*

Empathize as an Expression of Compassion

That tug you feel at your heart when you see a patient as vulnerable and suffering is called compassion. Your heart is speaking to the heart of another in need. Letting the person know that you see them as a real person in real discomfort is empowering to the patient. That simple connection may be just what they need to sustain themselves through whatever they are experiencing.

Embrace the Power of Presence: Listening and Touch

Touching is a touchy topic in our times, considering what some have endured. However, there is culturally acceptable touch. When I moved from New Orleans to the Midwest, I found hugging was one of my biggest challenges. I'd been living in the South for decades. There people hug, and it's not the sideways, arm-over-the-shoulder kind of thing. It's a real hug. In other parts of the country, people don't touch in the same way. In adapting to the local culture, I sometimes did (and still do) mess up.

Positive, healing touch can be a powerful presence. Massage and certain energy work have healing properties. However, merely a touch on a shoulder can be affirming.

Bear Witness

> *In your own Law it is written that the testimony of two*
> *people is true (John 8:17 NIV) .*

The art of listening is an essential element of healing on every level. Each time a story is told and then retold, the patient is processing the events and adapting to the new reality. Like the Psalms of Lament found in the Bible, listening to the story, sometimes again and again, is a way of bearing witness to the event and the journey. It is saying, "No matter how horrible it was, yes, this *did* happen." When we deflect the story or minimize it, we are relinquishing the honor of acknowledging the patient's experience. By listening, we allow them to find meaning as they reframe it.

One day in ICU, there was a patient who was to be transferred to the psych unit once she was medically stable. I went to see her, and my initial impression was that she was delusional. I wasn't sure what to do. One of my options was to get out of there in a hurry. But this was a person in need. What could I do without merely dismissing her?

She mentioned St. Bernard Parish, one of the worst hit locations in Hurricane Katrina. I asked her about her experience in what is euphemistically referred to in New Orleans area as "The Storm." The patient locked eyes with me and told me her story. It was absolutely heart-wrenching but, based on other storm stories I heard, not necessarily fantasy. There was a very good chance that what she told me had in fact happened. Her demeanor changed. She held her body differently. Her speech became intense. She shared her experience with me, and it resonated as true.

I really wanted not to hear the story. It was one of the stories that, once heard, something changes within you. I carry it with me still.

As I listened, I realized that perhaps part of her perceived mental problem was that she was still wrestling with the catastrophe more than five years later. Maybe she was trying to speak the unspeakable as a step out of reliving the horror. Trauma recovery can't be achieved alone. It is a collective process in which the pain is heard and witnessed and affirmed.

All I could offer that patient was my presence and support through intentional listening. My silent prayer was, "Lord keep me strong so I can hear this woman out. Lord, please give me the strength not to blink. Lord, use me to help this woman."

Could listening to her story make her well? Perhaps my value to that patient was simply to be one step in her journey. Perhaps not looking away and accepting her as a valued human being, no matter how broken she was at that moment, helped her in some way. To bear witness by listening and affirming is all I am called to do. To that charge I was faithful.

Simply being present, physically and emotionally, can be powerful. Each has its own energy. Each is important.

Confidence in Your Task

When I was working at EJGH, the General Practitioner residents followed chaplains for half a day as part of their training. The conditions of shadowing included that the doctor could not wear the white coat or the stethoscope. The residents had to shadow us as civilians without their power symbols. This provided a good opportunity for them to see what chaplains do, but also to enter the room and see the patient from a different perspective.

One day a resident and I entered an ICU room. The patient was sedated and on a ventilator. The adult daughter was sitting in the chair, reading. She smiled as I introduced myself and the doctor by our first names. As I was explaining that I was the chaplain, the pump started beeping very loudly.

Out of habit, the resident, who was stripped of her physician symbols, reached over and punched the buttons to silence the beeping pump. The daughter was alarmed. "What? Who are you??" She wasn't quite ready for the chaplains to manage the pumps. We smoothed it all out, but the image still makes me smile.

Offering

Offering is often associated with giving a financial contribution, particularly in church. There are other ways to consider the act of giving. *Offer* is a verb. An *offering* is a noun. So many nursing tasks are automatic. You enter the room and do a quick visual assessment. Then you glance at the monitor. It is easy to get lost in the busyness.

What if, in the midst of your busyness, you could pause? Make eye contact with the patient. Offer yourself through your attention to the patient. Your calming presence can be an offering. Holding a hand or offering to pray is a type of offering. These gestures are simple offerings to the patient. In the deepest sense, they are also offerings to God.

Spend time at the bedside, assisting patients in finding inner resources to sustain them in difficult situations. Help them find wisdom in that special in-between space where deep connection lies. Embracing that space can be beneficial to you as well as to the patient.

Points to Ponder

- What does spiritual care mean to you?
- In what ways might you be providing spiritual care already?
- What would you change if you could?
- What part of providing spiritual care is the easiest for you?
- What part of providing spiritual care is the most difficult for you?

...And You Might Try

What strength could you gain by saying a prayer for your day? It doesn't have to be complicated. Usually, the hardest part is just remembering to give it a try.

- Please, Lord. Help me through the day.

- Please, God, give me the words.

- Lord, give me strength.

If you aren't comfortable with prayer, consider a guided imagery where you draw strength, calm and comfort from higher power.

Remember, prayer need not be lofty in its ambitions. I pray for the person ahead of me in the express line at the grocery who has too many items and then needs a price check. "Please, Lord, help me find some good in this stressful situation."

Chapter 4:
Hospitality

*To be a fellow worker with God is the highest
aspiration of which we can conceive man capable.*

– Florence Nightingale (1973)

The hospital setting creates many opportunities to stand as God's presence, particularly in difficult situations. In the lingo of chaplains, *ministry of presence* means to be present and engaged as a form of service for God.

The change in a patient's status may be quick or slow. In the best possible scenario, the patient's pastor, rabbi, imam, or other spiritual leader is present with them, representing their faith community. However, often the chaplain stands with them in their chaos to represent comfort, hope, and God's witness as God's servant. Even more often, it is the nurse who holds that role.

A church's spiritual leader, often called a pastor or minister, is trained to lead a body of like-minded believers.

Chaplains do many of the same things as pastors, but they work in a nonreligious setting that is pluralistic and at times oppositional to church leadership. In *Outside the Walls*, Crick and Miller (2011, p. xiv) state that chaplains are trained in a practical theology that operates in "the muck of dysfunction, woundedness, and despair," beyond the walls of a brick and mortar church. In today's culture of declining church attendance, the chaplain may be the only pastor the patient or nurse has access to.

Smaller or rural hospitals sometimes rely on volunteer chaplains to fill the spiritual care gap. Frequently there is limited standardization of care or training. A sympathetic heart is one of many gifts that make a good chaplain, but cultural sensitivity and an appreciation of a diversity of faiths are critical components as well.

Often, the task of spiritual or soul care falls to the nurse. This is a challenging place to be because the work is intangible. It has to do with depth, value, relatedness, and heart – of the patient and of ourselves.

Some nurses are comfortable with providing spiritual care, and some are not. Working with the needs of individuals in the most intimate of settings may draw nurses to that role, whether intentionally or not. If the patient feels safe in the nurse's presence, that deeper Truth, the Soul, may step forth, speak its mind, and look for spiritual support.

Language as Common Ground

What is Truth? That's the classic question. In everyday context, truth refers to something that is proven. Your bank statement declares that you have $100.00 in your checking account. You withdraw $80.00 from the ATM, and the bank now declares that you have $20.00 in your account. That is micro truth.

When written with a capital *T, Truth* generally refers to universal or macro truth, meaning something that everyone holds true. For instance, gravity is held as a Truth because an apple falls from a tree no matter where it occurs on the earth.

There are common spiritual beliefs that are held as Truth throughout the world. Charity, love, and respect for others are Truths that form the bedrock of our everyday lives. These are examples of beliefs we share with our common humanity.

Just as we are all bound to earth by gravity, we are also bound together by an internal Truth that lies within each of us. It is the part of us that whispers in our ear to keep us from fooling ourselves about ourselves. That part of us, our core, is our spark of life, and it is called the Soul.

The Soul is who we are aside from our self-defined parameters. It is who we are when no one else is around. In it lies our connection to a Higher Power that major faiths,

Buddhists, Jews, Muslims, and Christians all refer to in terms of light.

Psychotherapist and theologian Thomas Moore (1992, p. xviii) describes the soul as the "font of who we are." The Soul is the part of us our ego can't control. It is the part of ourselves that wants to guide us to our highest good, before our ego steps in and shoves it out of the way.

Palmer (2009) uses the image of a shy child or a wild animal living in the woods to describe the soul's actions. Just because you may have decided to connect to the wisest part within you, patience is still key. The soul will reveal itself in its own time and space, and it is dependent on feeling safe and valued.

Listening in a Special Way

Hearing is the response to sound waves hitting and activating your ear drum. Listening is interpreting those sounds and assigning meaning to them. Within this context, we may designate different types of listening such as:

- **Active, or "Uh-huh" Listening."** For example, "What I hear you saying is…"
- **Sympathetic Listening.** For example, "That's really tough," or "I'm sorry to hear that happened to you."
- **Therapeutic Listening.** For example, "Tell me more about it…" or "How did that make you feel?"

These are the familiar tools that the nurse may apply regularly. Each has its own place, because listening is an essential part of professional nursing practice.

Another type of listening may not be so familiar, yet it sometimes makes its way into the conversation. It happens when we suddenly recognize there is a lot more going on than just exchanging words. Sometimes this realization comes in the middle of the conversation. That's holy time.

Lester: A Case Study in Listening

On a Wednesday evening in 2008, I was hard at work as a church pastor, preparing for a mid-week Bible study. I was scrambling around the parsonage, the house the church provides for the minister, preparing a new technology for our small rural church: *PowerPoint*. When a knock at the door interrupted my work, I groaned. I couldn't help it. It was too early for anyone from the parish to stop by. Since the house was on a main road, it could have been anybody.

At the door stood a large, older man. He was dressed in worn but clean overalls and held his ball cap respectfully in his hand. It took me a minute to recognize Lester, a regular customer at the church women's semiannual yard sale. Lester might be called a junk man. He'd buy some of the stuff that was left at the end of the sale to use himself or to resell to others.

He said he was thinking about coming to church, which is something people often say but rarely *do*, absent a personal invitation. I glanced at the clock, put a smile on my face, and suggested we go the few steps to the church office next door. Once there, we talked and made polite conversation in my office. I'm ashamed to admit that I kept one eye on the clock. I invited him to the evening study that was weighing heavily on my mind.

A part of me wanted to ease him out the door so I could finish my preparation, but another part of me was curious. What brought this large, awkward man, so dissimilar from the church's members, to my door? Something told me that I needed to stay in this situation and see how it was going to play out.

As we sat in my office, he gradually shared more of his story. He said he had been thinking of getting back to church for a while. But now he had incontinence problems, and he wasn't sure if he could make it through the length of the church service.

My heart instantly softened. I forgot the clock as I fully stepped into the conversation. My mind raced to find the words to reassure him.

I suggested we go into the sanctuary so we could figure out a plan. As we moved down the hall toward the front of the church, I pointed out the location of the restrooms. Maybe he would be comfortable if he could find a seat where he could slip out and go to the bathroom. As we walked, my mind focused on problem solving.

In the sanctuary, however, the conversation changed. My heart had opened to his. When I stepped fully into that moment of caring, he told me more. An almost imperceptible shift occurred in both of us. Lester had been diagnosed with a brain tumor. Surgery was an option, but not a guaranteed remedy. And that's when I got it. This man wasn't here about going to church; he was asking us to help him die.

It's hard to describe the sensation that washed over me. It wasn't so much fear, but more a feeling of caution regarding this subtle but powerful shift. For a moment, I was dumbstruck as I realized that this was why he had knocked on the door of the parsonage that day. It wasn't about me or the pretty windows in the nicely furnished church. He was asking for us to be with him on his journey toward death. At that moment, he and I were standing together in the presence of God.

That realization was powerful enough to scare me. A vivid image from the Old Testament flashed across my mind as I thought, "I see why they tie a rope on the foot of the priest." In the ancient days of the Jerusalem temple, only the High Priest could enter the most sacred place, the Holy of Holies, where God resided in the Ark of the Covenant. On Yom Kippur, the highest holy day, the priest would step behind the curtain, which hid the Ark from all but the priest. It was believed that if God was not pleased with the offering presented, the priest could be struck dead.

Since only the High Priest was allowed to enter the most sacred area, no one would be able to go in after the body. Only the priest was consecrated to stand in the presence of God. The solution was to tie a rope around the foot of the priest before he entered. Then, if he should die, his body could be pulled out.

I didn't have a rope tied to my foot that day. But as I stood with that large, awkward, rough-looking man in the middle of our North Mississippi church, I was certain we were standing in the presence of God. This happened only when I softened my heart to a soul in need and listened to his call for help. It happened when I listened – not with my ears, but with my heart.

Too Busy to Listen

How many times have I missed opportunities like this as I buried myself in busyness? That night, I had a PowerPoint projector to set up and important papers to run through the copier. I had lots of important stuff to do before Bible study.

What if I had asked that man to come back at a more convenient time? He wouldn't have. Parking his truck in my driveway and knocking on my door took immense courage. He said he had gone to every door of the church, and they were all locked. Coming next door to the parsonage was his last chance at connection. To be with a person when they are at their most vulnerable is an incredible invitation, often lost and rarely recovered.

In *Listening for the Soul*, Jean Stairs (2001) says that compassionate listening is intentional, intimate, and, in a broader sense, a form of hospitality. Hospitality? This is not a "setting out snacks and chilling down the drinks" type of hospitality. This is the ancient practice of welcoming a stranger as if God were present with you in the room.

Let brotherly love continue. Be not forgetful to entertain strangers: for thereby some have entertained angels unawares (Hebrews 13:1, NIV) .

Theology of the Heart

Jesus replied, 'Love the Lord your God with all your heart and with all your soul and with all your mind' (Matthew 22:37, NIV).

Theology is basically the study of God (or however you may refer to your Higher Power). Theologies are ideas about different ways to learn about God. Having a variety of ideas of God is good because it helps us find our own path. Along the way are a lot of choices and different roads to wander down. Having many ideas about God helps God find the way to reach us. God is always there. We're the ones who wander.

What part does God play in daily life? What are the beliefs inherent in each faith? Why does God want to be in a relationship with you or me or anybody else? These are the types of questions that come up around the topic of theology.

Here's a confession: the study of theology has never been one of my strengths, yet it is a part of who I am and how I do the work I do.

Another confession: theology gives me a headache. Personally, I would rather live my theology than discuss it, and I especially don't want to argue about it. Let me share my perspective. You can embrace it, or toss it out, or use it to help you think about your own thoughts of God. The important thing is to listen for the part that resonates with you.

For me, stumbling across a particular set of words in the book *Theological Reflection: Methods* by Graham, Walton, and Ward (2005), was a watershed moment. The words were: "Theology in Action, Theology of the Heart, and Theology in the Vernacular." At last, theology made sense to me! Finally, I could wrap my head and heart around how the study of God plays out in everyday life. I needed to find familiar words to help me define my God "boxes," and to capture the essence of what I do as a chaplain and as a Servant of God.

Theology in Action, Theology of the Heart, and Theology in the Vernacular are the way God and I work together. When I found those words, it was as if someone had read my heart.

Graham, Walton, and Ward provided me the language for what was an essential part of me, but one that I couldn't have described previously.

These three ideas explain a lot about my work in ministry outside the church walls, and they say a lot about me. In fact, when one of my spiritual directors retired, she gave a well-loved porcelain candleholder: an angel with a crooked halo.

She said, "Believe me. Many people have tried to straighten out that halo and it just won't." She told me it reminded her of me. Like the angel, I may get a little banged up, but it wouldn't take away my ability to share my light with others. Setting an intention to share our light with patients and families (the patients' families, as well as our own) can lead us to both professional and spiritual growth.

Points to Ponder

You may be more of a partner with God than you realize. Consider how might you act in the following situations.

Action: As you look over a new patient's chart, you notice that the drug dose as written could be taken one of two ways. Do you take the directive at face value, or do you investigate until you are satisfied with the answer?

Vernacular: You are present as the doctor gives test results to the patient. No family is present. The doctor quickly leaves, and you sense that the patient doesn't have a full understanding of what was just said. Do you leave the patient without explaining what the doctor said, or do you translate by putting the information in language that they can understand?

Heart: The patient in Room 14 is dying, and no family is present. How does your heart, your sense of compassion, respond as you provide care? Does it affect the patient's care?

...And You Might Try

If you have the time, think about your day as blocks of time defined by activity. Some blocks are longer; others are shorter.

Example 1: A call light goes on, and you go to respond to your patient. His pillow has fallen off the bed. You find the linen cart, go back in to change the pillowcase, and return to your desk. That's one block of time.

Example 2: The family member of a patient comes to the desk. She wasn't in the room when the doctor came, and she has questions. You update her, and she is satisfied. She goes back into the room. That's another block of time.

Think about your feelings in the two different situations. Are you able to distinguish these as separate units of time? Can you delineate the emotions that may come with each activity? Are your emotions as distinct as the actions involved, or do your feelings about one bleed over into the other?

Chapter 5:
Practice as an Art

Apprehension, uncertainty, waiting, expectation, fear of surprise, do a patient more harm than any exertion. Remember he is face-to-face with his enemy all the time.

– Florence Nightingale (2001)

The Art of Listening

"Caring must be enacted in order for it to be experienced and learned" (Bevis & Watson, 2000)

This morning, a bird was singing its song. It was throaty and full of life. As I listened, I was drawn into its beautiful tones. A part of me wished that I could sing along, but the song wasn't my song. Nonetheless, its beauty was true to the bird that was singing. Somehow, for just those few moments, I was drawn into the world of the bird, and it was a beautiful place to be.

Listening is a part of our everyday world. The jarring sound of a clock or phone tells us that it's time to come back from the land of dreams to everyday life. The coffee machine gurgles and hisses as it magically presents me with the gift of caffeine. Outside my window, I hear the noisy whoosh of the street cleaner, and I am relieved that I remembered to park on the correct side of the street last night.

To Hear or to Listen

The sounds are things I hear. They are noises that make their way down that elegant canal to hit my eardrum and activate the signals to my brain. Those sounds don't resonate with anything, save a quick thought about whether I have cream for my coffee. Hearing is different from listening. I hear the noise of the street cleaner. Putting the sound in a context of meaning is listening. Hearing involves the ears. Listening involves the heart and mind; you create the ideas that give meaning to what you just heard.

Listening is a part of every discipline. Nurses are coached on listening techniques, as are salespersons and customer care workers. Business, education, and nursing curriculums each emphasize the many types of listening.

1. **Active**... "Uh-huh" listening
2. **Sympathetic**... "That's really tough ..."
3. **Therapeutic**... "Tell me more about it..."

These are some of the standard responses, and they have their own place. But let's be honest. There are other ways to listen.

- **False listening** happens when we pretend to listen, but we're busy thinking of our own response.
- **Judgmental listening** occurs when we listen in order to evaluate, criticize, or otherwise pass judgement on what someone else says.

We Often Hear What We Expect to Hear

Here is a standard exchange.

Clare: *"Hello. How are you today?"*
Karen: *"Fine."*

But how would you react if the conversation went this way?

Clare: *"Hello. How are you today?"*
Karen: *"Oh, I'm so glad you asked! The water heater broke and flooded my basement. Then the door fell off the refrigerator and landed on my foot."*

The second conversation isn't what we expected to hear. It's not following the standard script, so it may be a little unsettling.

Most of the time, no matter how much we may intend to listen, what we hear is what we expect to hear. Our minds have a filter through which we experience life. Those filters are created by our knowledge, experience, and culture. When we challenge our standard expectations, the brain struggles to reclaim its familiar footing.

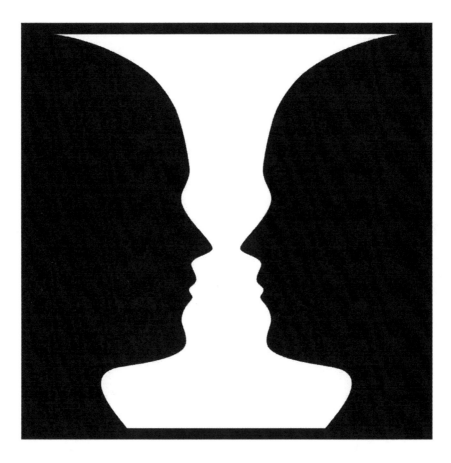

Image © Furian /Depositphotos.com, used under Standard License

This picture is an eye game. The same drawing can be interpreted in two different ways. At first glance, depending on how your brain interprets the picture, you'll see either a candlestick or two profiles facing each other. The brain comfortably picks one or the other. When challenged to look for the alternate version, the brain must shift to a different perspective. Our brains struggle to see things in a new way or to hear things in unexpected ways. We naturally resist struggle, taking the path of least resistance. That is why careful listening, not just hearing, is so important.

Careful listening is important to everyday life. You may hear a train horn nearby, but it is the listening – assigning meaning to the noise – that shapes your decision not to cross the tracks. Medical errors are often traced back to miscommunication, which can only be overcome by careful listening. Consider a situation in which the written prescription says one thing, and you hear the doctor say something else. Intentional listening is a habit that not only helps you maintain professionalism, but that also keeps your patient safe.

We often hear what we expect to hear. When that happens, we sometimes miss what is really being said. Our expectations are shaped by our own voices, prejudices, and opinions. An essential part of effective listening for nurses is the ability to set aside one's personal opinions and give value to what the patient is trying to say.

One nurse from my study said that she had an entirely different experience by becoming aware of her normal routine. She said, "The big thing has been an awareness of listening. If

I catch myself in a routine reaction, then I think to ask questions without interjecting myself into the conversation."

She said that she used to talk more about herself in response to what patients said, rather than listening and responding to them. She gave the example of one patient who worked in a profession similar to her father's. Normally, she would have attempted to connect with the patient through that commonality. But by asking a different set of questions, she discovered the patient's passion was raising horses. This opened to a deeper, more personal encounter with the patient.

"Now I do more listening and getting information. I catch myself more when I go back to the old way"
(Participant #9).

Listening as Relationship

Listening is about relationships. In a study of caring and professional practices, Vance (2003) asked nurses to describe patient engagement, or healing behaviors. The first four descriptors reported were touching, praying, caring, and attentive listening. Nurses clearly understand that nursing care goes beyond technical skills. The inclusion of prayer on this list, for example, reflects an understanding of the importance of the spiritual health of patients and their significant others. Inclusion of attentive listening as a healing behavior reflects just how central listening is to providing care. Again, the concept of listening is central to the care provided by nurses.

The relationship is two-sided, however. Just as the nurse listens and responds to the patient, the patient is reciprocating. The nurse questions and makes assessments, while the patient is doing his or her own assessment: "Is this someone I can trust?" Your actions, your bearing, and your attitude determine the patient's decision to trust or not.

Such scenarios aren't limited to the bedside. My study with critical care nurses included three short interviews and a longer taped interview about the use of the model that I taught. In one of my first interviews, I asked the nurse the survey question, "Have you noticed any change in your listening awareness?"

She looked me over. In nursing terms, I stood "assessed" on every level. Then, slowly, she responded. This was a nurse I knew well. It crossed my mind that she was deciding whether she was going to tell me what she thought I wanted to hear or trust me enough to speak her true mind. Once she appeared to make a decision, she looked me straight in the eye. She neither apologized nor showed regret for not engaging the process or even remembering to try it (Participant #13). Just like a patient assesses and decides whether to trust the nurse, the nurse I was speaking with decided that she could be honest with me. She deemed me safe, and she chose to speak her heart. That was a good thing for both of us. She maintained her sense of integrity about her participation in the study. I felt affirmed. I was honored that she trusted me enough to be honest.

Energy Fields

Our words are important, but what isn't said can be heard as well. In common language, we might comment on someone's "vibe" or "aura." That's the energy that we carry with us, and it is the patient's energy that we read or discern.

There is a bubble around us that defines our personal space. If someone stands too close, then we are uncomfortable because they are invading our private area. On the other hand, if we are holding our child or standing by someone we love, it can feel good to welcome them into our space.

We read the energy of others with our eyes, but also through our experience and our intuition, gleaned from years of patient care. How many times have you entered the room and known at first glance that something wasn't right with your patient? By the same token, the patient is reading you and your energy.

Bedside Energy

The ancient ones, those shamans and teachers rooted in vague history, say there is a force of energy that emanates from us, and that we carry around. This is why we are uncomfortable when someone stands too close. It is how we sense something is not right with a particular person. Your intuition that is grounded in your own space is speaking to you. As you can read others, others can read you. The thoughts you hold show your intentions and create an energy that can be picked up on, or read by, others. That's the part of listening that happens without using just your ears.

The space where interaction occurs between nurse and patient is special. Some may call it sacred. It is the place where both the patient and the nurse meet, bringing all of who they are.

For the nurse, it may be a conversation that helps clarify a situation. One of the study participants shared the case of a young mother who was physically disabled by her childbirth experience. The patient was first in ICU for some time and then transferred to the stepdown unit.

The stepdown nurse said that the patient had become very cranky with her caretakers. "You know patients can sometimes get mad at those who take care of them. I guess they figure we can't throw them out." The staff was concerned that the reality of her situation might be setting in, and there was discussion of a psychological consult.

The nurse wasn't satisfied. She sensed there was more going on, so through careful listening and questioning, she discovered that the current source of the patient's grief and subsequent behavior came from the fight between her family and the baby's father's family about who would care for the child.

The nurse said, "Can you imagine? It's bad enough when you can't even move your own pillow. She can't care for her own baby!"

The nurse spent time talking with the young mother. Once the patient opened up, they were able to talk about her feelings, and she listened and helped her process her situation (Participant #8).

The nurse felt compassion for her patient. Using the Quaker Listening Method gave her a path to experience what nurse theorist Jean Watson calls *transpersonal care* (2010b, p. 5). The mission of such care is to connect with another through presence in the moment as "authentic presence" (Watson, 2010b, p. 82). It is in these moments that nursing is more than a job. It is a call to a profession that is both life-giving and life-receiving, a profession that provides growth for a lifetime.

But Watson also notes that this caring moment can be taught and learned in theory. However, to fully understand its meaning, the moment must be experienced. Experience often brings understanding. The Listening Method herein described is a tool that can help open the door to this type of connection for nurses. As the hospital study showed, intentional listening allowed nurses to create the space for authentic connection with their patients.

It is one thing to understand the theory of transpersonal care. However, use of this Listening Method is compatible with the caring moment and provides a specific, practical method which may open the door for actual experience to occur. As the nurse's workload continues to increase, the inclination might be to avoid going so deep into the nursing experience. Don't dodge it. This connection can sustain and refresh your call to service. To be intentional means to focus and put your heart behind it. To be intentional means to fully connect and engage.

One effect of engagement is that patient care is improved. Yet in the process, we open ourselves to many possibilities for growth both professionally and personally. Our attention shows our intention to fully engage with another person.

Energy as a Ball

Imagine a game of "catch," in which the ball represents energy. Each of us has an unlimited supply of energy. Throughout the day, we are passing a portion of that energy back and forth to others. That is the energy impression that you pick up from others, even as you share yours with them.

In my experience, the energy usually appears as light. Sometimes it is strong, and people are drawn to it. On the other hand, sometimes the energy a person carries with them is dark or cloudy. As you push your cart down the aisle at the grocery, sometimes there are people you sense you don't want to get too close to. You can sense that without even looking at them. Something just seems off. If that energy were a ball, it would be like that person is constantly tossing out balls to see who might catch it. When you turn away, you are deflecting that ball and that vibe.

The ball toss is an invitation to engage. Remember, you don't have to play if you don't want to.

Every morning (and sometimes as I step into a potentially difficult situation) as I say my prayers, I place myself in an imaginary bubble of protective light. I call it the Holy Spirit, because that has significance for me. If you want to try it, you can call on the angels or use the name of whoever your Higher Power may be. I visualize myself in a cloud of white light. As I do so, I'm turning control of the situation over to that Power in full trust.

I also say that I'm doing this with no reversal on me or mine. If somebody is tossing balls of confused, negative energy at me, I don't want to be in a tennis game where we're hitting the ball back and forth. I don't want that energy to come back to me or to anyone I care about. It's an old method, but still a good one.

Jill Bolte-Taylor: Crisis Equals Opportunity

Just like the nurse assesses a patient based on knowledge, experience, intuition, and listening, the patient is using personal attributes to decide the degree to which they may want to engage with the nurse. This may come, in part, from an innate sense of self-protection.

Dr. Jill Bolte-Taylor, a Harvard neuroanatomist, wrote in *My Stroke of Insight* (2006), about her experience of having a stroke, recovering from a stroke, and what she learned in the process. When she was in her early thirties, she suffered a rare type of stroke that affected the language part of her brain. Her memories and ego stepped aside, and the immediate moment became the basis of her experience. Her filters were gone and with them, her memory. *Right now* was her only reality. A part of her brain remained engaged with her surroundings following the stroke. And, as a clinical professional, she observed her post-stroke care. One of her most profound reflections on her experience was her awareness of the energy that each person brought into the room with them.

From her experience, she came to identify that a hospital's number one responsibility is protecting the patient's energy levels – that is, what kind of energy is surrounding and supporting the patient's recovery. Positive or negative, the energy will affect the patient's response and perhaps even the ability to heal.

When I was a critical care chaplain working in the ICU, I sometimes sang to my patients when it was appropriate. One day an elderly man's blood pressure was labile, and two cardiologists watched the monitor outside his room. I didn't notice them at first and kept singing to the patient. When I emerged from the room, they were smiling. They said that as I sang to him, the patient's blood pressure stabilized. When I stopped singing, it became erratic again.

Patients are affected by the energy that is brought into the room. Bolte-Taylor (2009, p. 81) shared the story of a young female resident who "wanted to take something from me despite my fragile condition, and she had nothing to give me in return." She called the resident an "energy vampire." The resident was hasty and treated Bolte-Taylor roughly. "I felt like a detail that had fallen through someone's crack... [S]he insisted that ... I come to her in her time and at her pace, it was not satisfying for either of us. Her demands were annoying, and I felt weary from the encounter."

Later the same day, another resident entered her room. This doctor treated her gently and spoke encouragingly to her about her recovery, even though she was unable to respond. She said she felt acknowledged and safe, and his energy drew her out. She felt safe enough to "show up" for him and for his care. This challenges each of us to consider the energy we bring to the patient. Will the patient feel safe enough to "show up" for us?

Handling Your Energy

What energy you bring into the room is important for your patient, but it is important in other parts of your life as well. Imagine someone says or does something hurtful to you, just as you enter a patient's room. Maybe it's a snide comment, or perhaps somebody just rolled their eyes to imply you did something stupid. The very natural tendency is to react. Often we hold that reaction in and let it eat at us all day long.

"Well, I should have said…"
"Can you believe that?"
"I don't get paid enough to take that stuff!"

If you don't clear out that anger, frustration, or hurt, you carry it like a cloud that may not be physically visible but that can be perceived on every possible level. Like the *Peanuts* character Pig Pen, who walked around in a cloud of dust, you walk around with a muddled energy for the rest of the day. That is, if you let it cling to you that way.

After you leave work, who's going to bear the brunt of your energy? The cashier at the grocery store? The person who breaks into your lane? Your significant other? Your children? They may all catch the energy you lob their way!

Instead, shake it off. Take a deep breath, and imagine your negative feelings dripping out of your fingertips and dropping to the earth where they can be absorbed and transmuted into something positive. Physically stretch and let your body let go of what you are carrying wadded up in your muscles.

Another Kind of Energy

Consider for a moment the energy which is directed at you. Sometimes the energy is, good and sometimes it is not. I worked as a critical care chaplain for seven years. I had worked as an industrial chaplain for twelve years before that, during ten of which I concurrently served as minister to a local church in the deep South.

It's Not Always Personal

How somebody reacts says more about them then it does about you. I discovered that when I served as a church pastor. Often my interactions with the church members were as much about previous pastors or other authority figures as they were about me.

I had a series of confrontations with one church leader that I still struggle to understand. I represented something or someone to her that I was never able to overcome. The harder I tried to deescalate, the angrier she became. It worked out, though. That set of interactions led me out of the church and into full-time chaplaincy in New Orleans.

To be perfectly honest, some people just like to keep things stirred up. It is a form of entertainment for them, but they always have a self-righteous justification. In some cases, they have their own hurts and needs; they'll suck the life out of you, if you give them an opening.

Just because they ask, doesn't mean you have to engage them. Shake it off. Don't carry somebody else's baggage. I, for one, have enough of my own. I don't need to carry anyone else's!

Going Deeper

The idea of going to a deeper level of engagement with a patient might seem exhausting, but it is an invitation to reconnect with a part of you that may seem lost. What are the elements of burnout? There's a good chance you know them by heart. Exhaustion on every level, numbness, and detachment are all symptoms of a deeper problem. Burnout can disconnect you from the call to service that carried you through your training and sustained you for so long.

Asking questions and intentional listening can draw you into deeper communion with yourself and others. When we open ourselves up to the possibility that there are many levels of engagement, intentional listening at bedside may be one way that you find your way back to the nurse you remember once being.

*"I could see right there how just being open to where
they were and sometimes not saying a whole lot, but
just being open and listening, did a world of good"
(Participant #14).*

And why is that important? It's important because the
work you do is essential to who you are. It is work that calls to
you. It is something that you are. The life of service can be
sustained and even enriched when it is fully understood.

The Art of Healing

One of my friends is a critical care nurse. One day she
came by to dress my elderly mother's leg wound. Mother had
hit her leg and torn the skin a bit. Within a few days, the
wound became angry and weepy due to her advanced age and
ongoing vascular problems. She was on antibiotics and
required dressing changes. My friend stepped in to help and,
of course, did an expert job as she spoke with Mother, critically
assessing her every step of the way.

What happened next was even more profound. The whole
time she was attending to my mother, my big old grouchy dog,
Banjo, was on the other side of the room, licking a chronic sore
spot on her leg. The vet had told me that this would remain an
ongoing problem, since the dog was old, and there wasn't
anything to do for her.

My nurse friend glanced at the dog as she passed by to leave. She asked about the dog, and I gave her the vet's report. Her hand was on already the doorknob, but she stopped, let out a deep sigh, and turned around. She's a healer, and there was no way she could simply pass by a nursing need. She knelt next to Banjo and said, "Let me take a look at that." (She also said, "Don't tell anybody I worked on a dog!" For that reason, I have left her name out of the story.)

Amazingly, Banjo sensed she was safe in the care of this nurse. She allowed "her" nurse to examine her wound as closely as my mother's wound had been examined moments before. Banjo's nurse bound the wound so expertly that the dog couldn't get the bandage off for three days. When she finally got the wrappings off, the wound was healed. The "chronic problem" disappeared.

Banjo recognized a healing presence, and she trusted my friend to give her the support she needed to overcome a seemingly chronic problem. This is not just *what nurses do*. This is *who nurses are*.

The Art of Nursing

Nursing is an art. Those of you who are the healers are a blessing to the rest of us. Don't discount the power that you carry with you; it is your gift. Treasure it, especially as nursing becomes an increasingly quantifiable world. Numbers, measurements, and outcomes are part of a larger grid that seeks to find meaning in something tangible. Excel spreadsheets are comfortable because they can be printed out and held in our hands. Yet the soul of nursing speaks in another language that is discerned and then welcomed.

Florence Nightingale is remembered for establishing clinical practices that saved lives. What is often overlooked is her deep personal faith, which she revealed in her many writings. Her faith was the impetus that compelled her to elevate nursing to a profession. She believed prayer, love, and compassion affected the clinical outcome of patients. And she cautioned that compartmentalizing our personal and professional lives fragments care of self and of others.

Spirituality may be experienced in two ways. Individually, it is found in personal experience that may come through practices like prayer, meditation, or even spending time in nature. Spirituality can also be experienced communally, as people gather together to worship in a formal setting like a church, synagogue, or mosque. It can also be experienced in simple settings like at the bedside. In the Christian tradition, the belief is God can be present in every situation.

"Wherever two or three or gathered in my name I am with them." (Matthew 2:18, NIV)

Have you ever had a conversation with a patient that you felt was somehow "special"? Have you ever felt that your work involves something bigger than just yourself or the tasks that you do? Have you ever had a spiritual experience and discounted it? In that special time, you stood in the presence of what is often referred to as the Inner Teacher or the Soul. It is in those times of deep connection that Truth can find Its voice.

> *"The vent patient in #25 can't speak, but we communicate. Her eyes show me her response. I feel like we have a connection when I am intent on listening and remember the person inside the vent" (Participant #5).*

Palmer (2009) states that every time we gain through connection, each person is enriched. Admittedly, we aren't always successful in our attempts to connect on this deep level. But each time we try, we take a baby step. In time, we will connect with that Inner Teacher who waits for us to listen.

Our Wisdom, our Inner Teacher, invites us to move deeper to reconnect with our call to service by using intentional listening.

One of the nurses from my study responded to the question of whether she had used the new model she learned. She said that she doesn't rush to interject her stories into conversations with the patients.

"One day I thought, 'We all like to talk about ourselves, so why am I taking that away from my patient?' It's more helpful to keep them talking about them. The more information I can get from them, the better I can know and treat them. To understand them." She said the idea of listening isn't new, but she grinned and said, "I just never did work on it" (Participant #9).

Points to Ponder

Listening is different from hearing

- Hearing is a physical response by your ear to stimuli
- Listening brings meaning to those sounds through mind and heart

What does this mean for nurses and their life's work? ("Don't ask me to do anything else!") In the clinical setting, you are:

- Privy to the most intimate moments of life
- On the front line of patient care
- A symbol of trust

We often hear what we expect to hear. Our personal filter is shaped by experience, and our expectations can affect what we actually hear.

...And You Might Try

You are busy, right? What are you supposed to do with this?

- Realize the possibility that you may connect with others as they truly are, their Souls.
- Slow down a minute. Say a silent prayer if you are so inclined and know that the ground where souls meet is holy ground.
- Remember your call to the work you do and know that you are part of a greater good.

Chapter 6:
Bringing It Back Around

Nursing is an art: It is one of the fine arts: I almost said the finest of fine arts.

– Florence Nightingale (2019)

Somebody Else Gets It

One of the participants in my study shared a story in which an unrestrained patient was trying to pull out their ventilator.

"It just came to me. I saw myself in the bed and somebody coming toward me to tie me down. I wouldn't want it either. I don't blame them for being upset. The patient was confused and very afraid, and here was somebody coming at them with restraints... They kept yelling and fighting.

I was able to get through to them and explained to them what was happening and why...'If you don't fight it, then it won't be so bad.' Then I listened to what they were saying, and I helped them put their feelings into words. When they understood what was happening and why, they stopped fighting. In the past I would have just said, 'Sorry, this is gonna happen.' But then I took a minute and put myself in their place, and we didn't have to use the restraints. I felt we both won" (Participant #16).

"It just came to me." Somehow, the nurse was able to step away from her normal response to pause and see the situation in a new light. She connected to the patient through her heart. Listening with her heart affected her response. In the end, both she and the patient came to a mutual trust solution in a difficult situation.

John Wesley (1703-1791) is known as the founder of Methodism, a Protestant Church of which I am a minister. He is the author of *Primitive Physick* (2010), one of the most popular 18th-century books providing self-care advice and practical treatments for those who could not afford to see a doctor.

Wesley described special moments like the nurse experienced as a "Means of Grace," because it is in these moments that God draws close to be truly present and to provide insight. Visiting the sick, Wesley (2020) advised, is a means of grace because God is present.

When Friends Are More Than Friends

The Society of Friends, the Quakers, take the concept of grace a step further. For them, God is consistently present everywhere. So, for example, they believe there is no need for communion because God is present in every meal. Every meal is sacred. The sacred is present every day, in every way (Hamm, 2003).

Another Quaker belief is that if we wait for the appearance of God, God will appear through those who are around us. Within this context, their whole system of intentional listening is based on the belief that Wisdom lies within each of us and is ever present to guide us.

There is assigned practical wisdom that is gleaned from personal experience. Experience shapes wisdom as we reflect on actions and reactions that rise from it. As we reflect and weigh our observations, we assign them value. Wisdom is gained as we weigh those observations. Wisdom acquired this way could be called micro wisdom, as it is based on personal experience.

There is also a macro type of Wisdom, which is innate and sourced from the Soul or Inner Teacher, in the Quaker tradition.

Shortly after my younger son got his driver's license, he walked into the house holding an unfamiliar broken mailbox filled with someone else's mail. He had become the latest driver to hit a poorly placed, neighborhood mailbox that was often in disrepair.

"Mom, what am I supposed to do?"

"Robert, what do you think?" I asked.

He knew what to do. He was just hoping I would let him off the hook. He grimaced, got back in his car, and took the mailbox and its contents back to its rightful owner. The mailbox owner said that for all of the mailboxes he had lost over the years, Robert was the first to own up to being the guilty party.

This is our "Inner Teacher," who stands ready to help and guide us once we open ourselves to it. But it has to be invited. The first step is intentionally listening for its voice.

Some faiths call it God; others, soul. The Quakers call on spiritual companionship whether in worship, in business meetings, or in clearness committees.

Too often, the patient facing critical care decisions has come to the hospital following a slow decline. The family hasn't noticed the gradual change. The crisis appears to them as something sudden, rather than the result of a downward trend. Accepting the situation often takes time for the family to assimilate.

At this point, a nurse can step into action. A typical response may be to make a judgment on their situation and offer a solution. Using skills learned in the Quaker Listening method, however, can help the patient and the family to tap their own wisdom. A nurse does this through intentional listening and by asking open, honest questions. Intentional listening is expectant listening, similar to the waiting found in Quaker meetings.

An open, honest question is one:

1. To which the answer is not already known by you.
2. That does not lead. A leading question hints at the answer that you expect or want to hear. For example, "Did you go to counseling for that?"
3. That is neutral. "How did that make you feel?" A neutral question leaves room for the individual to respond in any way. There are no inherent expectations.

Therefore, an open, honest question is one that cannot be answered with a "yes" or "no" and one whose answer is not known in advance. This type of question opens the door to connection, inviting wisdom to step forth and participate in the medical care discussions.

One day, I stood as a member of an industrial chaplain team on the belly of a half-constructed oil rig. Around me sat hard working folks who stopped to eat their supper. Lunch boxes, paper bags, and thermoses of hot coffee were scattered around them on the floor. For those who might be interested,

I shared some positive thoughts about God. It was then that I first came to appreciate Wesley's boldness of theology-in-action, in bringing the God's Word to those outside of the church walls.

As a white, female clergy wearing steel toed shoes and a hard hat, this site was foreign to me. Similarly, Wesley had left the church pulpit to stand in an open field and preach to a thousand people. This congregation was more comfortable hearing God's Word outdoors, than sitting on a hard bench in a cold church. It was something that he never thought he would do, but he assessed the situation and acted to fill a need. That sounds like a nurse to me.

Yet in being God's presence to those pipe fitters and welders, my heart was touched by their individual needs. Through my interactions with them, my ministry was formed. I was probably changed more by them than the other way around. I came to realize that coming to people where they are physically, emotionally, and spiritually was the Theology in Action, which is also known as praxis. Graham et al. say that praxis in theology is "performative knowledge" (p. 170), which means that our knowing and our doing are inseparable.

Theology-in-Action / Praxis

The roots of praxis are biblical. Praxis is about Jesus when he "entered the temple area and drove out all who were buying and selling there. He overturned the tables of the money changers and the benches of those selling doves" (Matthew 21:12, NIV).

The theology of Jesus included a belief that an unjust situation requires a response. Praxis is a familiar idea in nursing. For a nurse who is responsible for the care and safety of the patient, this concept works within the parameters of both personal and professional ethics.

Theology-in-action is a term that developed from the work of Brazilian educator and philosopher Paulo Freire, whose writings (1968) on the oppressed deeply influenced education and theology. He focused on emancipatory learning, or seeing things in a new way, as a means of transformation. His focus was on the politically oppressed, but I believe this idea is compatible with the ministry at bedside.

I watched as families wrestled with end-of-life decisions. So often it was like the patient was sustained – or one might say *imprisoned* – unconscious, on life support. Sometimes the patient lived in that space between full life and full death for weeks. It was demanding for the patient and their family, to be sure. And it was often stressful for the nurse, trained to save lives, to provide what was essentially futile care. At times in the hospital setting, the patient must be emancipated from poorly made health decisions by the family.

Praxis is a basic element of nursing. Emancipatory knowing is one of five ways of knowing taught in nursing, and it centers on sharing power and responsibility (Smith-Stoner, 2011). Other elements of this knowing are awareness of context and the social factors surrounding patient care. Twenty-first century nurses are coming into complex healthcare settings that require advocates for vulnerable patients, who often are unable to speak for themselves.

The nurse's primary responsibility is patient safety. Relieving or freeing the patient from psychological, physical, and spiritual suffering is a cornerstone of nursing. Florence Nightingale's lifelong commitment to improving the state of medical care in Britain is emblematic of this biblical hospitality nursing in action, as is the image of her walking the halls with a lamp, checking on Crimean War injured in her care.

The Quakers exemplify theology-in-action as well. Their deep commitment to social action and peace is well documented in their peaceful protests over the years (Quaker Information, 2019). The basis of this action is simple: all activity is sacred. The Spirit of Christ, or the Inner Teacher, lies within each of us. Respect must be given to all.

Accessing the wisdom, or what they call the Light within, is available to anyone at any time, from corporate worship to an assembled Clearness Committee or other form of listening for the soul. Anticipation acts as an invitation to the emergence of the Inner Light. One element that delineates the Quaker Listening Method from other listening models is the Quaker concept of Wisdom as a change agent. Wisdom, or the Soul, can make itself known, even in the midst of the anxieties of patients and families in health crisis.

Theology in the Vernacular

When they heard this sound, a crowd came together in bewilderment, because each one heard their own language being spoken (Acts 2:6, NIV).

Theology in the Vernacular as described by Graham, et al., is theology based in the familiar. Vernacular is particular to a specific time and place, where the boundaries lie within accepted language and common symbols. It is fluid, not static, and responds to the current culture.

This is like code switching, which is responding to the immediate situation and switching between languages midstream. For example, code switching occurs when a multilingual person switches between two languages as needed. One day on a hospital elevator, I overheard a conversation of a Hispanic family. The child spoke to one woman in English, and to another woman who appeared to be her grandmother, she spoke Spanish. I was caught up in the rhythm of the language as the girl slipped back and forth between the two women, responding to them in the appropriate language.

Individual English words like "email" popped up in the conversation like popcorn hitting a hot skillet. Code switching can be a survival skill, a cultural identifier, or something as simple as a high school kid who slips from one way of speaking to a friend to another as he addresses his teacher. Think about how, in a work setting, you may speak one way to your peers and another to a patient.

Holy Spirit: A Case Study

In 1999, I was a chaplain intern at a Baptist hospital in Jackson, Mississippi. A chance interaction with a patient showed me that God not only comes to us in our greatest need, but also communicates in a very clear language of the heart. As I entered the hospital room to visit a patient, I passed a doctor who was leaving. Inside the room, I found the patient and her husband sitting quietly.

The visit was awkward. After all, this was twenty years ago, when women were not always welcomed as clergy. I felt that I had not connected with them on any level and assumed it was something I said or did. I spoke a few words, offered a prayer, and was relieved to get away.

Later that day, I was called back to see the patient again. I winced and dragged my feet back up to the patient's room. I didn't see the point of going back, but I went anyway. Imagine my shock to discover that the tension I felt earlier in the day had nothing to do with me!

The doctor I passed in the doorway had just delivered the worst possible news. They were still in shock as they tried to take in what he had said. They remembered my visit, which was why they asked me to return.

The patient and her husband said that I had said exactly what they needed to hear, and that my prayer was exactly what had been on their hearts. The voice may have been mine, but there was a greater presence there with us. It is in the most difficult moments when hope may seem elusive, that we need God most. Yet in those moments, God stands closest to us through the presence of the Holy Spirit.

The Walk to Emmaus Was More Than a Stroll

That moment with the patient reminds me of the unrecognized Jesus, breaking the bread with two disciples, in the gospel story of the walk to Emmaus. Two disciples walked with this stranger and shared their greatest sorrows. Little did they know that it was Jesus with whom they had shared their broken hearts, following his crucifixion. In the breaking of the bread, the disciples came to see the truth before them as they recognized Jesus.

When he was at the table with them, he took bread, gave thanks, broke it, and began to give it to them. Then their eyes

111

were opened, and they recognized him, and he disappeared from their sight. They asked each other, "Were not our hearts burning within us while he talked with us on the road and opened the Scriptures to us?" (Luke 24:30-32, NIV).

Fr. Dominic Maruca, SJ, calls this "walking in faith together" (2019), as we act as spiritual companions to others. He says it is like a Third Presence that comes and falls in step with you. Maybe that person shares his or her life, and you hear about their suffering. Things often fall into place. As you look around, you can see you have shared something remarkable with that other person.

When asked whether she had experienced any difference in her own spirituality after learning this new Listening Method, one of the nurses in the study said:

"Yes. By that I would say that this model promotes a universal way of experiencing God. By that I mean that I am opening up, and it is easier to see God in others. I've become more aware and I sense that sometimes the Holy Spirit gives me the right words for that patient. Especially this last patient who wasn't exactly spiritual or religious. I especially felt it there" (Participant #14).

In some faiths, this is called the presence of the Holy Spirit. In the Quaker faith, it would be considered the presence of the Inner Teacher providing the Wisdom specific to that situation. I soon realized that, with Wisdom's participation, there are always enough people present to form a Clearness Committee, no matter how many or how few are in the room.

Points to Ponder

- Have you ever considered how your personal view of spirituality might affect your patient assessment?
- Do any of the three models below speak to you more than the others?
  - Theology in the Vernacular, or everyday speech or presence
  - Theology in Action, or taking up a cause you believe in
  - Theology of the Heart, or feeling moved to act on the behalf of another

...And You Might Try

Practice using open-ended, honest questions. Here are some examples:

- How did that make you feel?
- Why do you think that happened?
- What does that mean?
- How did you think it would turn out?
- What did you mean by that?
- How did that work for you?

- And the best one of all...   Would you care to tell me more?

Chapter 7:
It's Pretty Basic

So never lose an opportunity of urging a practical beginning, however small, for it is wonderful how often in such matters the mustard-seed germinates and roots itself.

– Florence Nightingale (2019)

Listening is not a passive act. It requires energy and engagement and is an essential part of good communication, which in turn affects patient care and safety. Medical errors are often traced to miscommunication. Patients report that they feel they matter when the nurse listens to them. That can affect the hospital's bottom line. Listening is an essential art of intentional nursing care.

Attentive listening as a healing behavior reflects the basic essence of listening in providing care. Varying types of listening skills, such as Active Listening, are woven throughout the current nursing curriculum. With Active Listening, we hear the words of the other, process the information, and then use our response to structure further discussion. A phrase often used in Active Listening is, "What I hear you saying is..."

The patient assessment includes reading the patient's response on every level, verbal and nonverbal, and it is a fundamental part of nursing. It is important, however, to remember that hearing and listening are two different things. Hearing occurs when sound hits the eardrum and it vibrates. Listening makes meaning out of that sound.

The nurse's assessment is anchored in knowledge that comes from formal education, both personal and clinical experience, intuition, and listening. Each of these is shaped by our expectations. We see what we expect to see. We hear what we expect to hear. And as the nurse gleans information from the patient, the nurse's personal filter affects how that information is processed.

When asked if using the listening model affected care, one nurse said, "Working with patients, [the model] allows me the chance to place myself by using listening skills, by using empathy, to place myself in their situation. And therefore, I become more in tune to hearing and to listening and to seeing what they want. So I can better understand their situation" (Participant #16).

Listening in a New Way

Have you ever noticed that when you wear a new pair of shoes, you are more aware of how you walk? As your heel touches the ground, your weight shifts within the shoe to accommodate the new way it is forcing you to walk. Your foot wants to go to its familiar gait, but the new shoe says, "No." Walking is calling for your attention. Suddenly, you are stimulated to engage your walk in a different way. You become aware. You are tuned into your steps as your body accommodates something new and different.

Listening in a new way can be like that too. It can be like the new shoes that require your attention, instead of the comfortable old ones that you slide on without even having to tie the laces. Deep listening requires you to tune yourself to the nuance that is often hidden in the message. One of the study nurses described how patients often are indirect in getting their message across and reflected upon the responsibility that comes with searching for their meaning:

> *"Because the folks don't always say directly but they can kind of imply that maybe that's how they would deal with a situation. So you have to listen to what they are saying and not try to get them to say what you want them to say or what you think they need to say or in that way but to really listen to what they are saying and then feel comfortable with the message they are giving you even*

117

though it may not be a direct as you would put it if you were in their place... You have to truly listen. It's challenging" (Participant #2).

What is Attentive Listening? What is Deep Listening?

There are different levels of listening. The image of an onion is one way to visualize different levels of listening. The outside layer is dry, brittle shell that can easily be slipped off, because there is no connection to the life that originally grew it. Regular, everyday listening is sort of like that. The dry outside skin is only one slight layer deep, easily sloughed off and tossed away. Watching TV can be like that, too. As I drank my coffee this morning, I heard ten or fifteen commercials, but I can't repeat back to you a single featured product. I heard the words of the commercials but there was no takeaway message. Hearing is like that. How many times do we listen and nod and say, "Uh-huh," without connecting on any significant level?

Once the first dry layer slides off the onion, we find a new and different experience. A scratch of this layer reveals something moist and pungent, something that feels like it has a little more life. It is attached to the rest of the onion. Here's a connection. Just picking it off from the rest of the onion can make you cry. That second layer is connected to those below. It is good and can be chopped up to add a little zest to the soup.

But an onion is not a one-trick pony. Take a knife and dig deeper. With each additional layer, the flavor is stronger and offers more possibilities. Roasting an onion yields a much different result than sautéing it. Each technique adds unique flavors and textures to your finished product. Application is the key.

The same goes for listening. Interaction with a patient can be as dry and lifeless as the outer skin of an onion. Or it can be savory and rich. It's your choice, and that choice is influenced not only by your intent, but by the circumstances around you. Staffing, charting, and all kinds of roadblocks will inevitably pop up; yet your intention is the guiding light.

As one nurse explained her experience:

"So we really need to just stop and open up space and just sort of clear the air to let them express what they need to express. Or to work through the things that are on their mind. Because reassuring them all the time doesn't work. You know, you can tell them over and over, 'You're going to be fine'...That doesn't alleviate the worry that they have. All the questions going through their head are still there" (Participant #12).

The nurse curriculum offers many listening techniques, so one may wonder why another one is necessary. Many of the standard methods of learning are like that first, sloughed-off skin of the onion. They don't require much of the listener. Scratching the next level of listening opens the door to opportunity to better connect with your patient. As one nurse said, using the listening model helped her in "opening up a human connection," as she called it (Participant #12).

"We're all on this earth trying to work things out, right? We're all a part of something bigger. It's good when we can go deeper into the conversation" (Participant #12).

Remember, there is a difference between hearing and listening. Hearing is simply taking in sounds without any interpretation. Listening calls on all the senses and especially the heart.

The "Ting's the Thing"

The Chinese have an ancient symbol that presents the basic elements of intentional listening. The symbol is called 'Ting.' There are several models of this symbol, but the one used within my study included listening not only with the ear, but also with the eye, undivided attention, and the heart.

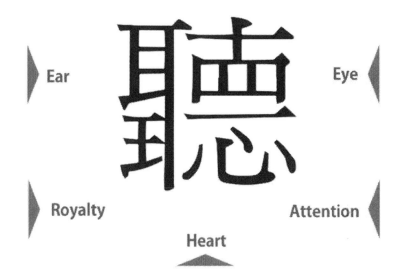

The large symbol represents attentive listening. The smaller symbols that comprise it represent elements of good listening. Combined, they express that listening involves the whole body of the listener. This is what happens when you shed the dry, outer skin of the onion and travel a layer or two deeper, as you connect. Instead of getting distracted, Ting helps us to pause, to focus, and to choose – to listen more intently. And it only takes a moment.

Elements of Ting

Ears

Listening with the ears may seem obvious. Many times, though, we hear what we expect to hear or what we want to hear. The same is true for patients and their families. One of the study nurses commented, "Being more aware of my listening has made me more open to asking about the patient's perceptions." The nurse said she feels like she's really listening to what the person is saying, and doesn't just say, "uh-huh..." and wait for them to finish (Participant #1).

Your Engagement

A warm body does not engagement make. The decision to be focused and present is essential.

Attention / Intuition

Fire burns hot. It draws us towards it. We like the feel of the warmth, but our senses tell us when we get too close. There is a play of give-and-take. Too close. Too far. Conversation can be like that too, and we need our intuition to read the situation and honor the other person's space. Our intuition tells us if we are standing too close or if we need to inch closer. Perhaps we even sense if the person needs a touch on the shoulder, or to have their hand held.

Wisdom stands with you in the room and speaks to your intuition. When we listen to the wisdom within the interaction with another person, then we will be guided to what is needed for the moment.

"I focus on what the other person is actually saying. I really listen to what is being said. I make sure that what

is being said is understood. And I stop what I am doing,
I look at the person, give them my total attention and I
listen to them and I also listen to myself... what my self
is saying. And I just listen" (Participant #3).

Another nurse described what happened when she was not fully attentive. She said the family came to withdraw treatment. When the family asked how the patient was doing, the nurse responded to their questions, but the information totally threw off the family.

"I have to give them the truth. That's my job, but I should have listened to their body language more," she admitted. "If I had engaged them a little more before I blasted them with the truth, then it would have been easier to hear it from me... I should have gone to them, rather than pulling them to me. I wanted them to go in and see her, but they wouldn't enter the room."

The nurse and I discussed what that represented to her. She said, "I read their mom one way... you know, professionally. They know her better than I do. I guess I wanted them to confirm what I was thinking about the patient" (Participant #14).

Eyes

One of the project's survey questions was, "Did you feel any connection with the person as you used the model?" The nurse's response was that she definitely felt more connected to the patient as she used the model. She talked about a patient she had the week who was embarrassed that she could not control her bowels:

> *"I was reading her and not just hearing her words but reading her body and her facial expressions. I told her that accidents didn't matter. I didn't mind cleaning her up. But, of course, what I said wasn't going to put her at ease. She was going for a CAT scan and was worried she might have an accident in there. I realized I was more careful in my listening and in asking her questions. She was really appreciative. I told her that we would work out something for her, and it seemed to bring her comfort. It was like I was listening and responding to her on a lot of different levels" (Participant #14).*

Eyes are as important as ears when it comes to deep listening. Sometimes a person says one thing, but their actions say something else. Their actions don't resonate as true. Or as my then four-year-old son once asked my sister, "Can I borrow your ice cream cone?" The eye can catch the subtleties.

Heart

One day I came into an ICU room where a young man, awake and alert, was waiting for swelling to go down so he could have back surgery. I introduced myself as the chaplain, and he immediately began talking. He said in a soft Louisiana drawl, "I don't get it. Y'all don't know me. I think I'm kind of intuitive. I feel like everybody who walks in here comes with love in their heart."

Listening with the heart means listening compassionately and without judgement. Compassionate listening is a gift to yourself and others that sometimes gets lost. "Compassion fatigue" is a well-documented effect on anyone who is working in a high-stress situation. It is expressed as physical and mental exhaustion resulting from exposure to a traumatized person (Cocker & Joss , 2016). Working with higher levels of acuity patients, increasing demands of the job and of personal life, can drain a nurse's well of compassion. That is why self-care is so important. Rest, time for reflection, and debriefing after tough cases can all help to replenish the proverbial well. When we are in a personal space where our hearts resonate with suffering, we share what it is to be human with another. Intentional listening can be an important part of this process.

One nurse said that careful listening helped her with difficult patients, and that her awareness helps her to think about what their perceptions are. "They're in a hard spot, and sometimes I just need to stop and look at things their way. I think this helps me be a better person especially with difficult people." She mentioned a relatively young man on the floor who was on a vent and not likely to get off. "I felt like he knew

I was trying to communicate... that I cared. That felt good" (Participant #1).

Royalty

Some of the written versions of Ting, the Chinese character for listening, include one more symbol: royalty.

Our modern-day perception of royalty is shaped by what we hear and see on the news, or by the storybook weddings we find in fashion magazines. In the old days, royalty exercised sovereign power over their subjects. Whatever the king commanded was carried out. If the king commanded you to go to war, you left everything and marched off to war. Since royalty held the power over your very life, listening was critical.

In this discussion of listening, we use the word *royalty* as a reminder to treat the one speaking as if they are royalty, which means listening with respect and honor. True listening treats the other person as if they are someone important, someone special.

One of the study nurses shared the story of the man who kept raising his bed to a dangerously high level. She went in to see what the noise was about, because the staff was telling him the bed had to come down to a safer level, and he loudly disagreed.

The nurse went in to explain that his settings violated hospital policy. He again argued for the bed height. He told her that he is a very tall man, and the bed was a little short for him. The lower bed height made him look up to watch TV, which strained his neck.

She said, "I put myself in his position to see why he was doing something so crazy." When she saw his height, she understood and stopped to think of a solution. She was respectful, but still found a way to compromise (Participant #16).

Where to Start?

A question is an invitation to listen. Communication on every level is the cornerstone of listening. As you assess a patient, what is it you are doing? As you are running down your checklist, you are asking questions of your patient, but you are also asking questions of yourself. Your questions show the patient that you want to hear what they have to say. When a patient asks a question, treat it as an invitation to step into their life.

Remembering to Remember

Habits are hard to break. This is a well-known fact. Remembering to remember to listen was one of the biggest challenges for each of the study participants. After admitting in the first of three interviews that she kept forgetting to use the model, one of the study nurses found some value in using the model.

She shared her experience on a recent trip to the eye doctor when she wasn't wearing her contact lenses. Since she couldn't see well, she was more aware of how many people came in and out of the examination room without introducing themselves. She said it was irritating to not be able to make out their faces or to know who they were. Careful listening came to mind. She used the analogy of contact lenses and hearing aids. "Listening in a new way is like seeing with enhanced contacts, or in this case, enhanced hearing aids. It's just better" (Participant #13).

Living with Intention

Remembering to listen intentionally is the key. Is there possibly a trigger to help you remember? What is something you do on a regular basis that you could use to help you remember to listen more intently? Little gestures or reminders can help.

I use the ritual of the hand cleanser. Before I enter the patient's room I stop, take a breath, pump the cleanser and rub my hands, and go in. Others include these steps and add one. Think of your feet as deep roots going down into the earth to ground you as you release the previous patient, before you step in to meet the next one. Just those few seconds can help you break from the previous activity. It is like a minibreak. It is a small but effective method of resetting my intent, so that I'm not burdening the next patient with whatever happened immediately before I see them.

Two small steps can make a big difference.

- Refresh with a breath, and
- Reset with an intention to be more present with the patient, family member, or staff person.

Take a breath and set your intention. To be intentional means to fully connect or to engage.

One of my study nurses shared how her intention became fortified by something she saw on the news following the shooting of children at an Amish school. The wife of the man who shot the children knew nothing about the husband's plan, and the men of the Amish community came to her home and reached out to her in a gesture of peace and grace.

The next day at her husband's funeral, the wife was frightened for herself and her daughter as the press rushed to her car and yelled questions at her. As she pulled up in front of the church, the Amish men again appeared. This time, they surrounded her and her daughter to shield them from the press and allow them privacy. "If those men can do that, then I think I should be able to stand and listen and be present for people in tough situations. I am going to do that" (Participant #2).

Standing tough with the person in your care, being that person's advocate and protector, is part of the higher call in nursing. Certainly, it can help with the hospital's survey scores, but there is something more at stake. Your sense of personal integrity, how you feel about what you are and what you do, is what is important. And as you stand with and for your patient, you open yourself up to the many possibilities for growth, both professionally and personally. Our attention shows our intention to fully engage with another person and sets the stage for authentic relationship.

The Survey: Listening

The traditional medical model of physician-centered care is shifting to that of patient-centered care, as reflected by the Medicare survey of patients following hospital admission. The Hospital Consumer Assessment of Healthcare Providers and Systems (HCAHPS) patient survey provide the basis of millions of dollars in Medicare payments to hospitals. The Hospital Value-Based Purchasing (VBP) Program, part of the Affordable Care Act, now requires that the percentage of hospital reimbursement be based on core quality measures, including the HCAHPS patient survey.

"During this hospital stay, how often did nurses listen carefully to you?" This is the first of 27 questions on the HCAHPS survey. Perception is everything, and if the patient – or the significant other who fills out the survey for the patient – does not experience relational contact with their nurses, the hospital's bottom line will suffer.

The Survey: What's Not Covered

Technology gobbles up time and elbows out the personal interaction between nurse and patient. The nurse's eyes, previously used to scan every facet of the patient, now remain fixed on the tablet screen, as the assessment becomes a series of established questions to carefully place the patient into a larger algorithm, all dictated by insurance billing. Numbers are important.

The heart of nursing does not lie in technology. Holistic care requires care of the patient on all levels, including emotional and spiritual, as well as physical. Holistic care reflects a move away from technologically centered care, often referred to as modern or traditional medicine. This transition has contributed to the new emphasis away from the historic doctor-driven patient relationship, toward that of patient-centered care. However, the challenge is that technology is often at odds with holistic care, which is hard to quantify.

The Medicare survey sent out to patients following a hospital stay measures *patient-centered care*. Recall that the very first question is, "During this hospital stay, how often did nurses listen carefully to you?" What would be your score on the Medicare survey? If it were your patient answering the survey, how would you score?

Points to Ponder

As you are assessing the patient, they and their family are assessing you. They are asking themselves, "Is this somebody I can trust?"

Intentional nursing is about compassionate care and that includes the art of listening. This is listening in a NEW WAY. Remember: the Ting's the thing!

...And You Might Try

Remember to remember. Intention shows your willingness to engage.

Before you enter a room:

- Take a breath
- Set your intention
- Prepare to engage

Chapter 8:
Down the Garden Path

Were there none who were discontented with what they have, the world would never reach anything better.

– Florence Nightingale
("Oxford Essential Quotations", 2016)

"Caring responses accept person not only as he or she is now but as what he or she may become. The potential of a person is as important as the person in their current state of being."

– Jean Watson (2008)

Listening: Scratch or Dig

Let's go back to the image of the onion to consider levels of listening. The "uh-huh" type of listening is much like white noise or the dry skin of the onion. There is no meaningful connection to the rest of the onion, and it is something sloughed off before you get to the "good stuff." It is here, and then it is gone.

The next level is like scratching the first ring of the onion. That top level is serviceable. It can be chopped up or even fried. The twang that hits your nose reminds you that there is life in that top ring, and that life is sustained by the connection to the rest of the onion.

The Chinese symbol for Ting reminds us first of what constitutes deep listening, which includes listening not only with the ears, but with the other elements as well. Our eyes pick up the non-verbal cues. Our attention confirms our intention to listen fully, and in the process, it activates our intuition as well.

The importance of listening is universal.
The Chinese language symbol *TING* expresses all elements of listening.

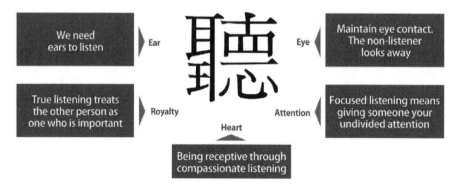

We need ears to listen — Ear

Eye — Maintain eye contact. The non-listener looks away

True listening treats the other person as one who is important — Royalty

Attention — Focused listening means giving someone your undivided attention

Heart

Being receptive through compassionate listening

These elements help us scratch our way through that top layer of listening that is a step beyond the dry, onion skin, "half-listening" type of listening. In a way, they represent transitioning from hearing to listening, because they are the gateways to the person with whom you seek deeper interaction.

But we have only scratched the surface. The other elements of Ting: heart and royalty, are an invitation to dig even deeper, to go past that first ring of engaged listening as we invite some emotional elements of the heart. Remember, we hear with our ears; we listen with our hearts.

That sounds like a good phrase, doesn't it? But what does it really mean, and how does it work? How can it be a part of spiritual care? And, by the way, who has time? And... How do you even begin?

It All Begins with a Question

Questions are essential, and they are integral to spiritual care. The last time you were with an unfamiliar group of people, you probably started the conversation with a question like, "How have you been?" or "What's going on?" If you are talking with a stranger you might ask, "How do you know...?" or "Where do your kids go to school?"

As the conversation unfolds, it builds upon asking a question to which the other person responds. Then, they ask questions of you. The conversation flows organically as each of you exchanges questions and statements.

It is not that much different when you are working with patients. Think of the questions you ask every day.

- **Level I - Dry, onion-skin type of question:** "On a scale from one to ten, how would you rate your pain?" This can be a springboard type of question, that can open the door to further communication. Or not. It's up to you to choose.
- **Level II - Next layer of the onion:** The response to that question can draw you to another level. "Has there been a change for you?" This is where Chinese Ting type of listening can be applied, as you listen not just with your ears, but also allowing your eyes to read body language as you begin to give the patient your full attention.
- **Level III - Getting down to the deep, pungent center of the onion:** This level involves listening not just with your ears, eyes, and attention, but also with your heart. It requires responding with open, honest questions such as, "How is that working for you?"

Spirit will bring questions to you as you make your way along your spiritual path. One of my favorite discussions with my children occurred on the long drive to the Gulf Coast of Florida for a beach vacation. My younger son was asleep in the back seat. My older son (who would grow up to become an Episcopal priest) was about eight years old. The road stretched out before us, and things got deep fast.

"Why am I here? What am I supposed to do?" he asked me. Those are good questions, aren't they? I've asked them for myself even as a grownup. Over the miles, we talked about God and paths of life that open up for each of us. That time together with my son was sacred space as we spoke about bigger concerns than just our everyday life. The same thing can happen between you and a patient at the bedside, between you and other staff, or between you and a beloved family member.

Sometimes Asking Questions Requires a Little Push

I had to push myself to ask more questions when I became a chaplain. Amongst the things I learned growing up, I had always been told that it was impolite to ask personal questions. Indeed, if I were too curious about somebody, I would get a stern look or a swift kick under the table. I had to overcome my reluctance when I first entered chaplaincy. I felt asking questions was an intrusion. Maybe you had a similar upbringing to mine.

We must remind ourselves that questions indicate interest. If too few are asked, it feels as if something is missing. Recently I spent the day with someone new at work. I had never met him before, and there were long stretches in the day where we were sitting around waiting for something to happen. Within a pretty short time, I knew that he was married, had two girls (and their ages), how he met his wife, and where he went to school. And what did he know about me? He only knew the information that I volunteered on my own. He didn't ask questions of me but seemed happy when I asked about him and his life. I don't know if he wasn't curious about me, or maybe he was just being polite. But the lack of questions made me feel that he wasn't interested in coming to know me.

Questions are integral to the spiritual path because they tug us along as we go. A question calls us to go deeper.

Listening with Both Sides of Your Brain

Remember Bolte-Taylor, who suffered a stroke at the young age of 37? One morning her mind stopped working, and she was thrown in a world that she had studied as a Harvard brain scientist but had never experienced. While her brain was in the process of stroking, a part of her remained the scientific observer. I am frequently reminded of the distinction she draws between the "energy vampire" and the other resident who engaged her through his words and kind presence.

Bolte-Taylor's book, in fact, opened my eyes to the energy fields around us, and an awareness of the energy I bring into each patient's room. However, it was her 2008 TED Talk, in which she describes the two hemispheres of the brain, that provided me an "Aha!" moment. There is plenty of information on the left/right brain connection, but her presentation helped me to put into words something I had been wrestling with for a while: explaining the personal shift that can result in providing spiritual care.

Bolte-Taylor's talk may stir some memories from your basic anatomy class. In her TED Talk, she exhibits an actual human brain, which clearly demonstrates how the two halves of the brain really are separate from one another, connected only by a slim middle part called *corpus callosum,* through which signals are constantly passing back and forth between the two hemispheres.

The right brain thinks in pictures, or what she calls the "collage of the present moment." The right brain is filled with sensory experience that connects with the world through feelings and senses like sounds and tastes. It is the right brain that connects our energy to that of the world around us. The right brain is the "we," which is the connection we share through energy. It is the collective.

The left brain thought process is linear and orderly. It takes the information from the right brain, categorizes the information, and assigns meaning to it. This is the home of "brain chatter" which, in effect, anchors us to the external world through organization. Bolte-Taylor demonstrates that the left brain takes the right brain information, categorizes it, associates it with the past, and projects that information onto the future. The left brain is the seat of "I am," the place where we identify ourselves as separate from others. Personal identity, the "Me," detaches each of us from the greater flow of energy around us.

Our left brain, that inner chatter that constantly speaks to us, is where most of us live. We see ourselves as rugged individuals who can stand alone and manage crises big and small. This is especially comfortable for those of us who depend on our minds, critical thinking, and resourcefulness to provide care for our patients throughout the day.

A garden analogy comes to mind. Imagine two separate but equal gardens that sit side by side, separated by a fence. On one side, you'd find a neat and tidy vegetable garden, with linear rows and carefully printed names on posts beside each of the well-tended plants. This is like Mr. McGregor's garden in *Peter Rabbit* (Potter, 2008). Everything is orderly, well maintained, and has its place. This is the left brain.

The flower garden on the other side of the fence is strikingly different. In fact, it more resembles a jungle like in Maurice Sendak's children's book *Where the Wild Things Are* (1988). This lush garden is filled with bright flowers and rich aromas. The flowers and herbs spill over their boundaries and blow gently in the wind. The vegetation is unrestrained. This is the right brain.

The gate in the fence separating the two gardens is unusual in that it freely swings in either direction. The corpus callosum, that middle section where information passes constantly between the gardens, is much like a bee gathering pollen from either side. The mind selects what information it needs from either side as needed.

Each side has its comforts. The left-side vegetable garden is organized into neat sections by type and color and carefully weeded. Imagine standing with rake in hand, admiring how well cared for and tidy this garden is. Everything has its place. Order can be refreshing.

On the other side, the flower garden is filled with colors and smells and sounds. Abundant flowers in every color are everywhere. Blue morning glory vines wrap around tall stalks of sunflowers. Encompassing peace fills the space. Taking it all in has us swimming in a sea of connectedness with something bigger than ourselves. Some may call it a Higher Power. Others may call it God. This is the place of deep connection to everybody and everything.

To take it a step further, imagine the orderly well-tended garden as being the personality. It is who you present to the world, and it is all that establishes you as an individual or the "I." It represents the past and the future.

The wildflower garden, grounded in sensation and the immediate moment, is the part that feels the energy of self within a greater sea of connection. This represents self as we seek to connect to a bigger context of energy. This represents the "we."

The We Connection: We Are a Part of Something Bigger, Whether We Like It or Not

While we generally envision ourselves as separate individuals, we stand in unity with all sentient beings. Stand too close to another person, and we invade their personal space; it is a collision of energies. For a more complex example, consider attending a football or basketball game. Those who fill the stands share a common spirit of wanting their team to win. This is shared energy.

My first year at EJGH hospital was the same year that our "home team" took home the biggest trophy in professional football . I was on call the Sunday of the semi-final game. I completed my rounds early that day, because I knew no one would want to talk after kickoff. Later, as I was stepping off the elevator, something dramatic happened in the football game. Someone must have fumbled the ball, because there was an instantaneous, collective moan from patients and staff. The noise poured out of the rooms, rolled down the empty halls, and echoed throughout the whole hospital. That was a hospital filled with individuals standing in unity and shared energy. It was a palpable experience.

Standing at the Gate

Imagine again the two gardens, separated by a gate that freely swings back and forth like kitchen door at your favorite restaurant. In watching the wait staff as they move easily back and forth between the dining room and the kitchen, a natural rhythm emerges.

The brain responds in a similar manner. Left brain and right brain are in constant communication; the right brain picks up images and sends them over to the left brain to be categorized. If the corpus callosum that stands between two sides of the brain is like the garden gate, imagine how many times a day that gate swings back and forth. The flower garden records undefined impressions, and the vegetable garden categorizes them and gives them names and meaning.

What does gardening have to do with being a well-skilled clinician? Imagine the garden gate as the door to your next patient's room. As you enter the room to do your assessment, you step into the left-brain vegetable garden. Order is created as you react to impressions and complete your assessment. Questions asked. Questions answered. As they are answered, your mind is observing, categorizing, and placing the answers into tidy rows. You fit the responses into anticipated outcomes.

What might happen, though, if you were to pause as you stand at the garden gate? You look to the flower garden and consider going on a different path. You know the left brain well and all that the vegetable garden represents. Maybe something is calling you to scratch the surface and to go just a little deeper.

Why? The longing for deep connection that the flower garden represents is calling to your heart. Connection is what brought you to nursing in the first place. Connection is the source of deep satisfaction. And it is in connection that you can be refreshed and restored.

The Special Space

Remember yesterday when you came home from work? What is your routine? Many homes have a porch or mud room or even entry hall. You opened the door and came in. You put your keys down and maybe took off your shoes before you fully entered the house. There was a physical and emotional transition from the outside world to inside your home, allowing you to relax and enjoy your personal space.

Commercial spaces and churches also have transitional areas that bridge the outside and inside spaces. Churches have a narthex or entry hall. Office buildings, doctors' offices, and even hospitals have lobbies and waiting areas that provide for areas of similar transition. Some consider that the halls of the hospital are also such a place, as the patient transitions from a place of wellness to that of care or cure (Pigott, Hargreaves, & Power, 2016).

Think about the last time you went to the doctor. You entered the office, signed in, took a chair, and waited. You were not outside the office, and you weren't fully in the examination rooms. You were in an in-between space that is neither here nor there.

In those seemingly calm areas of transition, you have time to catch your breath and center your thoughts before you go on to the next step.

Spiritual care lies in those in-between spaces where one is not fully rooted in either space. It is the gate between the two gardens. It is also the space that lies between the business model of bio-medical healthcare and the mystery of the human condition. The "in-between" space, often called "liminal," may be difficult to grasp because of the quantitative mindset of the medical professions. There is no familiar language, no formula to describe where mystery lives.

For Bolte-Taylor, her stroke placed her in a liminal space that enveloped her. It beckoned her to remain in the warmth and peace that she called "La La Land." It was such a wonderful place to be that she had to struggle to keep one foot in the "real world," so she could fight for her recovery.

That is one attempt to describe the indescribable. In many faith traditions, this is where Soul or Teacher, the wisest part of ourselves, resides. Accessing this liminal space and applying intentional listening provides one model for communication for this unquantifiable world of *Soul*.

Our desire is to be part of something greater than ourselves. What we do is foundational to who we are individually. The call to nursing is not about self, but about service to others. That call to serve, to put someone's needs before our own, calls to us. Nursing is the type of work that calls to you. It chooses you to live in a particular way, learn complicated skills, and then express your concern for others through your actions.

Ultimately, this desire is about love. The dictionary tells us of all types of love, but it is the selfless, unconditional love for God and others that the Greeks named *agape*. This type of love, love for others as we are loved by God, sustains the selfless deep care and connection that a nurse holds for his or her patients. One nurse explained it this way:

"You know, nursing is a great profession. You touch people in a way that other professions you don't have that opportunity. You can really make a difference in their life and have an impact on their life and that experience can be positive for the family. That's such a strong and positive thing" (Participant #2).

She went on to tell me about a letter she received from a patient's family following the patient's discharge. The family commented on how meaningful one nurse's care was to the patient. The letter testified how supportive care can directly affect patient outcome:

[The family] said the nurse really helped create a turning point in the recovery because of the way she supported them with her expertise, her peacefulness, her reassuring manner, all of those things really made a difference in that they really saw this as a true calling from her. And they were really happy and benefited from having her care for them. So ...nursing is a great opportunity to do all of that (Participant #2).

Jean Watson and the Caring Moment

Nurse theorist Jean Watson created a nursing model based on the recognized value of both the nurse and the patient. The foundation of care emphasizes the common connection between caregiver and patient as each seeks to connect and embrace the soul of the other (Bevis & Watson, 2000). It is a yearning that seeks connection. This is expressed not only in the process of caring and healing but through authentic relationship within what she refers to as a Caring Moment. This moment, that special connection at bedside, is like one link of a chain that was first forged eons ago when one person reached out to care for another. The links of that chain wind their way along the healing journey, from a beginning that begins in some primordial haze, continuing through time until today. You are one link in this chain. It began before you, and it will continue long after you are gone. You are part of a great tradition.

This Caring Moment is anchored in compassion. Compassion is from the heart. Empathy can create a reaction within, but compassion is a little different. Empathy reflects a desire to understand another's emotions. It resonates with the brain and the body. Compassion comes from the heart, as it motivates us to caring *action* to relieve the suffering or discomfort.

In that moment, your heart resonates with another's, and there is a desire to respond in some manner. Fully listening and engaging with your patient provides an outlet for the emotion that wells up inside. Actionable compassion, like a wave hitting the shore, carries you forward to deep connection.

Points to Ponder

Is it possible that all through the day, your body responds in ways you might not even recognize? Take part of your shift and become aware of your body.

- Someone stands close to you. If it feels good, then you've let down your guard and allowed someone into your space.
- If it does not feel good, then maybe you sense energy that isn't compatible with yours. That's someone invading your

personal space. Perhaps it is like that energy vampire Bolte-Taylor describes.

...And You Might Try

Notice how many times during the day your body speaks to you.

- Perhaps you hesitate at the door before you enter a patient's room. Suddenly there is heaviness in your chest, and your feet feel glued to the floor
- Your patient says something to you, and you feel a twinge in your heart.

Each of these is a physical reaction to a visceral experience.

Chapter 9:
The Model

*[T]he symptoms or the sufferings generally considered
to be inevitable and incident to the disease are very
often not symptoms of the disease at all, but of
something quite different...*

– Florence Nightingale (2019)

The Quakers, or Society of Friends, have a 400-year-old Listening Method, which taps into the wisdom of the Soul. It is a unique way of listening that is often used in difficult situations. Questions like "Should I change jobs?" or "Do I really want to get married?" require careful examination. The first step is asking a question specific regarding the topic at hand.

As you may recall, an open, honest question is one that:

1. You don't know the answer to
2. Does not lead
3. Is neutral

Let the response to the first question guide you to the next one. Stay on task, and only ask questions about what the person wants to explore.

One day I became acutely aware of how this was working for me. Following my interviews with my nurses, I was trying to glean overall themes from what my nurses shared with me. I didn't want to create boxes that I could fit their responses into. Instead, I wanted to truly understand what they were saying and draw a few simple conclusions from their words.

I sat in my pastoral care office at the large hospital where I worked, wrestling with this question for a while. My director began asking me a few open, honest questions.

- "What look did the nurse have on her face as she responded to the question?"
- "What is the thread in responses to that particular question?"

With help from an ongoing discussion throughout the day, I discerned circular themes of intentionality. That is, the intentional use of the model, care, experience, and spirituality. My director's thoughtful questions encouraged me to tap into a greater wisdom. My process was allowed to unfold once I let go of my need to somehow "corner my results." In other words, I let reflection and intuition help me find the nurses' voice in the process.

Listening for the Light

The Quakers' holistic belief in the unity of all persons, at all times, is compatible with the nature of today's healthcare setting. The belief is that the Spirit, Soul, or Inner Light, exists within each person and is available for inner guidance. This inner wisdom has its own perspective and offers choice through its guidance, which comes through expectant, intentional listening.

Expectant listening is an effective model of discernment that has proven itself over centuries. Palmer (2009) notes that while Inner Wisdom is completely reliable, it is not easy to tap into. Discussion of soul work, after all, is rarely a part of everyday conversation. Inner Wisdom is not easily accessed because it is shy, much like a child introduced to strangers. Asking open, honest questions indicates interest and helps promote a sense of safety, inviting the quiet Wisdom to speak.

When someone in the Quaker community has a personal question to decide, they may choose to call a group of people together to help discern the best outcome. This group is called a Clearness Committee. The person presents the problem, and then the committee ask questions only about the topic at hand. In the right setting, the committee can help an individual find that inner teacher that is consistently reliable as compared to the culture around us. Also, the committee acknowledges that we need people to help hear that wisdom, and to recognize that voice from within. To listen like the Clearness Committee is to listen for the Wisdom within. Have you ever noticed patients often ask questions, not necessarily for information, but rather to confirm either what they know already, or what they think they know?

Often people don't listen because they are busy planning their response. Or perhaps they rush into the conversation and interrupt or cut the person off. Often people rush to fix, even if they aren't asked to do so. Many times, there is miscommunication, and the conversation becomes personal with hurt feelings ensuing.

Clearness Committee

The Basic Premise

We each have wisdom within, which the Quakers call the Inner Teacher. We need other people to listen and help us access that wisdom. The committee welcomes and seeks to support the presence of the Seeker's Inner Wisdom. It is invitational listening. The Quaker belief underscores that God is present in every facet of life. Remaining open to this Higher Power as an active participant is an essential element of the committee.

The Format

The structure consists of a few friends and associates who come together by invitation of the person seeking to find a solution to a particular question. There are certain elements, corporate and individual, that are basic to participation in a Clearness Committee.

Corporate

The basic elements include an invitation by the one we could call the Seeker. That is the person who is seeking an answer to a question. To be invited implies the Seeker trusts the participants, this being essential to establishing a feeling of safety.

There is a preselected topic of discussion. The Clearness Committee knows beforehand what question the Seeker is attempting to answer. Questions are limited to the problem at hand, so the entire Committee can stay on task. There is also a common understanding that a specific solution may not be found immediately; rather, this may be one step in the Seeker's journey toward the best outcome.

Individual

The focus is on the Seeker and on the individual's process of tapping the Wisdom within. It is important to ask open, honest questions specific to the question at hand. Questions are limited to that which the Seeker is trying to resolve. For this reason, it is essential not to interject oneself into the Seeker's process. Statements like, "The same thing happened to my Uncle Joe," are distracting and pull the focus away from the Seeker, toward the one who made the statement. These statements contribute nothing to the solution.

Patience is essential. There should be no rush as the Seeker is allowed time to work through their process, in their own time and in their own way. Just like a wise person doesn't step out in the middle of traffic, Wisdom takes its time to make itself known. The Committee allows the Seeker enough space to do the work at his or her own pace.

A Clearness Committee may be part of a bigger process for the Seeker, and that is something the participants have to trust. Although the meeting may end without a specific resolution, the Seeker may still be processing. As part of trusting the Seeker's process, it important that participants don't mention the meeting unless the Seeker does. It's like avoiding the temptation to take the lid off the saucepot too soon. Simmering is as valid a method of cooking as using the Jiffy Pot. Each cooks at its own best pace.

Can this model be used in a clinical setting?

Stepping back and looking at the Quaker Listening Model within the context of transpersonal nursing, the answer is "Yes!" An essential element of the Clearness Committee is neutrality or being non-judgmental. Watson (1980) posits that a nurse can empathetically communicate without conveying judgement. The model can be used one-on-one, nurse-to-patient, as the patient works out a question. You, the nurse, can be like a Committee of One. You establish trust as you offer yourself and not your judgement. This work takes patience because you can't just call out the Wisdom. It has to find the courage to speak up. Your patient is not the only one asking, "Is this somebody I can trust?"

Primary commonalties between the Clearness Committee and Transpersonal Nursing include:

- Belief in a higher spiritual force within each individual
- Change may occur through intentional or expectant listening
- Meaning can be found in the shared moment
- A caring, safe environment is essential

It Starts with a Question

A question is an invitation. Think back to the simplest of questions, "How are you?" A question opens the door to interaction. An open, honest question is one that closes the door on an easy answer like "yes" or "no," which can shut down the conversation.

An open, honest question is neutral, and one to which you don't already know the answer. Questions such as "How did that make you feel?" or "What did you think when that happened?" do two things. First, the person cannot dismiss you with a simple "yes" or "no." Second, you are indicating your interest by inviting the other person to respond.

If this sounds complicated, remember it is the patient who opens the door to this type of communication. The patient has intuited that, as you stood at the garden gate, you were willing to dig deeper into the rich garden of the right-brained "We." When the patient asks a question, it is an invitation to go deep. Be willing to find the richness in this caring moment.

The next part is the hardest. It is waiting in the tension as the Wisdom within the person gauges whether it will "show up." Remember how Jill Bolte-Taylor trusted the supportive resident who treated her with respect. Once she judged him as trustworthy, she decided to "show up," to pull herself out of her fog, and engage him. That was a big step toward her healing.

An acronym that might help you remember the waiting part of the process is the word **SAT**.

- **S**it indicates your presence.
- **A**ttentively indicates your engagement.
- **T**rust indicates your belief that the Inner Teacher is present and vitally active in the discernment process.

It is a tough place to be in, but don't blink. Stand in the quiet; from the tension, often the best answers bubble up. Sometimes, just as we rush to fill in the quiet space, Truth emerges. But nurses are caregivers who want to solve the problem! In controlling your deep-seated temptation to "fix," you are allowing the patient to do their own work. This is powerful.

As humans we like to give our opinions. But this is a time to, as the old saying goes, "hold your tongue." And that includes afterwards as well. When you see the person again, don't bring up the topic, because you don't know where they are in their process. Maybe they've reached some type of decision. Maybe they are shy that they spoke to you.

The Committee understands:

- There may be no resolution at the time of the Committee, but one may bubble to the surface later.
- This may be only one step in a person's process.
- It's in talking things out that solutions are often found.

and

- There is a bigger process going on than just merely exchanging words or conversation. Respecting the process and acknowledging the presence of the Inner Teacher can lead to the deeper connection.

Another aspect which may be difficult, is that you may never know the resolution. The answer to the question or challenge may bubble to consciousness much later. Think of links in a chain. Your part is to be patient and to be faithful in your intent to help. You can be satisfied that you have done your part. Trust in the outcome. Believe in the possibility.

Working with the soul is, as Palmer says, like trying to make friends with a shy child (2009). Wisdom will make itself known when it feels safe and isn't rushed.

How Do You Start? Who? What? Why? When? Where?

When is it appropriate to use a model such as this? Consider the basics. A question is an invitation. At times, the hospital staff is called to provide what chaplains refer to as a "ministry of presence" – not only to patients, but to family and staff as well. The simple act of presence is powerful. Using a tool like the Quakers' intentional listening model is a gift of service. And in reconnecting to that deeper Self, both sides of the equation — nurse and patient — are enriched.

How do you start? It begins with intentional use of the listening model.

- **Who:** Patients or families who ask you for your advice
- **What:** Open, honest questions
    - Ask question that you don't know the answer to
    - Don't ask 'yes' or 'no' questions
- **Why:** To help person find the truth from within
- **When:** To be asked a question is an invitation to help them find their answer

- **Where:**   Any place that feels safe

Trust the process. Perhaps there isn't a resolution now, but trust that the process is working, whether it is obvious or not. An answer may bubble to the surface later. It is in talking things through that solutions are often found.

Get ready. If you consider yourself a trained listener, you may assume that listening is something you can handle well. Consider this. What would be your response if right now, as you focused on a task, someone interrupted to ask you for your advice. What would be your immediate response? Would you hesitate before offering an opinion? Would your mind nimbly run through a thousand solutions as the question hangs in the air? You may think you know, but often what we think we would do is very different from what we end up doing.

Things Aren't Always as They Seem

In a recent NPR.org podcast, "Hidden Brain," science writer Shankar Vedantam presented studies that discussed what is called the "Hot/Cold Empathy Gap" (2019). The studies show that our logical self can effectively outline a plan of action ...that is completely lost once we are in the middle of strong emotions such as anger, fear, or sexual arousal. Our strong emotions disconnect us from the logical side of our brain.

Vedantam uses the example of the comedienne Morgan Smalley, who left her venue following a stellar performance. She hit the proverbial ball out of the park that night, and she was basking in the glow of the perfect evening.

A man approached her with some random items in a shoebox. There were some pens, an Amazon gift card, and a pair of shoes that weren't even her size. The man said he'd sell the box to her for $25. She laughed and said sure. After all, she was on a roll!

Even though it was dark and late, and she didn't know this man, she took him to her ATM. She could only withdraw cash in twenty-dollar increments. She asked if he would sell her the stuff for $20. When he said no, she withdrew $40, which she gave to him for a shoebox full of items, most likely stolen from unlocked cars. She later justified her behavior to her family, "But he was such a nice guy!"

In her aroused state following her great performance, she completely lost track of her logical self.

It happened to her. It can happen to you.

We may think we can handle it, but that is our cold logic speaking and not our hot emotional self. The emotional self reacts automatically, despite our best efforts. When our emotions are heightened, we can lose our calm self.

A Solution

It may seem impossible to overcome a seemingly automatic response. However, the studies also proved that the most effective solution to being on autopilot was training. It is possible to override our seemingly automatic reactions by learning a different response. The good news is that, just as in acquiring any physical skill, muscle memory can be changed. Anticipating and practicing a different response to intense situations can change how you respond.

There is a 400-year-old Listening Method that can help create a new response to the sudden life questions. It can provide an override to your usual response as you shift the attention back to the other person and away from you. And in the process, you can help them find the best solution: the one that they find for themselves.

It all begins by asking them a question.

Points to Ponder

As I settle into the conference room, I perch uncomfortably on the arm of the sofa. I look around at the assembled group of family, nurses, and medical staff, all gathered together for a family meeting. It strikes me that this scene could play out as easily around a kitchen table or an ancient campfire.

There is power in sitting with others in a circle, and it reminds me of scripture.

> *For where two or three come together in my name, there am I with them (Matthew 18:29, NIV).*

With this in mind, I realize that no matter how many or how few are present, there are always enough to form a circle (or a Committee) to help someone grapple with life's big questions.

Remember:

- The model is a tool for helping people find their own solutions, not yours.
- The format to use is question-response-question.

...And You Might Try

Try practicing your open, honest questions so that you are ready when situations come up. You might experiment as you go about your day.

When a co-worker shares that they watched a movie with their family, ask, "What was the best part about that?"

If your child comes home after a tough day and complains about the amount of homework still to do, ask, "When your friend didn't sit with you at lunch, how did that make you feel?"

When the clerk at the grocery store asks you if you want your bag to be paper or plastic, ask, "What do people usually get?"

That last one is a stretch, I admit. But this is a challenge to "think outside the box." Asking a thoughtful question is a counterpoint to our habitual responses, which often close down a conversation before it begins...

"How are you?"
"Fine."

Where can a conversation go from that point? Deep listening can lead to deep connection. Deep connection can lead to transformation. It all begins with a question.

Chapter 10:
Steppingstones

Every nurse must grow. No nurse can stand still. She must go forward or she will go backward every year.

– Florence Nightingale (2015)

"I was very interested and…it really just clicked. Everything clicked. And it was something I guess that I had been trying to change in myself for a while, so it just kind of brought all that together and put it into words."

– Participant #10

What Did Caroline Do?

It had been a long shift already. Why does it seem so many things come to a head at 3:00 a.m.? Two thirds of the way through her shift, Nurse Caroline stood in the doorway of Room 4, anticipating the question that would come next. When the call light rang, she knew what the patient's wife was going to ask her.

What would you do if this were your family?

Caroline had her own opinion about the patient's condition. This patient's trajectory has a seemingly inevitable end. The easiest thing to do would be to give her opinion and continue her duties. Caroline had come to know the patient's wife and considered her a level-headed woman. Over the course of admissions, the wife had come to trust her. She felt it.

The listening model the chaplain taught her wasn't about the nurse solving the patient's problem. It was about helping the patient and loved ones use their own resources, as they make their way on this part of their journey. What if, instead of offering her own opinion of the patient's condition, she tried this new listening model. Is it possible it could work?

How would you handle this situation? Is it possible to come up with a different scenario?

A Listening Sample

It all begins with a question.

[Scene: A hospital room. A nurse enters the semi-dark room and does a quick assessment as her eyes adjust to change in light.]

Nurse: Hello. How's it going?

Wife: He doesn't seem to be getting any better.

Nurse: He seems stable for now.

Wife: (sighing deeply) What's next?

Nurse: What would you like to happen next?

Wife: I'm not sure. I wish he could just be fixed so we could get out of here.

Nurse: Have you and your husband talked about what the next step might be?

Wife: We kind of talked about what was important to us. How we wanted to live out our days. But we always talked about it as a couple. You know. Being together. We've been together for over forty years.

Nurse: When you talked about it, what were the important parts? What makes for a good quality of life?

Wife: Being with family. Being together. Golf was always important to him. Having that time with his friends. He hasn't been able to do that for a long time though. That's been a big loss for him.

Nurse: So within his limitations, what would be the best life he can have?

Wife: I think keeping him comfortable is what's most important now. Looks like this might be the best we have for a while. If he's home, the grandkids can be around more. I know he misses his dog. The dog misses him.

Nurse: Is having him at home something you can handle? What kind of family support do you have?

Wife: Our kids live close by, and they are good at coming by and giving me a break. My sister just recently retired. She's a nurse. I don't want to have to depend on her completely.

Nurse: So, you've got good support. If you could bring him home again, is that something you would want to do?

Wife: He always said he wanted to die at home. He hates coming to the hospital. He feels so isolated from his life. Maybe the best thing is just to do what we can and take him home.

Nurse: When you say that out loud, how does it feel?

Wife: I didn't think I was ready to accept that we were at this point. Somehow saying it makes it more real. But putting it into words feels a little better.

What did this interaction provide?

From the nurse's perspective:

1. The nurse showed that she was willing to engage fully in the conversation. She was focused fully on the task of listening. Her attention showed her full intention to engage in the conversation.
2. She didn't rush the conversation, but let it open organically.
3. The nurse did not solve the problem but led the wife through a series of questions that were specific to the problem. As she stayed on task, the wife was able to consider her resources. As she did so, new ideas came to her. The nurse did not lead the wife to a solution but helped her access the wisdom within.
4. The nurse did not distract from the conversation by suggesting solutions or by interjecting herself into the conversation. She didn't lead the wife in any direction but allowed the wife to direct the conversation through her responses.
5. There was no direct resolution, but the conversation helped clarify her situation and got her thinking in a different direction.

From the wife's perspective:

1. The wife trusted the nurse and felt safe asking difficult questions.
2. As she responded to the nurse's questions, she clarified the situation for herself.

171

3. The questions helped her remember conversations with her husband, which in turn helped her consider her options.
4. The questions empowered her to create a new plan for her husband.

The nurse in this scenario had come to know the patient over a series of admissions to the hospital. But even if this were his first admission, her heart could resonate with his situation.

Deep listening leads to deep connection. Deep listening can also be an expression of compassion. Listening is an easily accessible response to that resonant heart. Compassion calls us to action. Actionable compassion, applying action in response to that tug to the heart, is empowerment.

One of the study nurses stated that a young father's situation really spoke to her heart. A young father who had been very ill missed his home life. In particular, he wanted very much to see his very young daughter, but he was afraid that seeing him in the hospital setting would scare her. He confided in the nurse, "I don't want her to see me on these machines."

The nurse said that through use of the listening and questioning model, she assisted him as he worked out his need to see her and his concerns for her possible long-term response. Through the conversation, he decided to postpone the visit until he was in a less intimidating setting. The study nurse said that listening was an essential part of the patient's process (Participant #9).

Memory as Refreshment

Remembering the "why" of your nursing practice can sustain you through the toughest of times. It may help you remember that heart resonance that drew you to this profession. For me, it is remembering my Uncle C.H., who lay at home for seven years in a coma and my Aunt Frances' plea, "Why didn't the doctor say something before we put in the feeding tube?"

For you, it may be remembering a special patient or a family member you helped. Each of us has something that keeps us going. Remember and be refreshed.

The participants in my study reported that intentional listening provided three basic outcomes on personal nursing practice.

1. Enhanced empathy
2. Increased personal report of spirituality, which meant at times they were aware of the presence of God in their work
3. Improved communication

One of the younger nurse participants in my study said that while listening is talked about in the nursing curriculum, practicing the model helped make listening easier. She said that the Quaker Listening Method is compatible with the listening methods taught in school, and that it has helped her become more intentional about taking the time to listen (Participant #4).

Intentional use of the model worked for nurses in my study, and it can work for you. The hardest part is remembering to use it. The hardest part is to change your routine.

Points to Ponder

"It is when we include caring and love in our work and our life that we discover and affirm that nursing, like teaching, is more than just a job, but a life -giving and life -receiving career for a lifetime of growth and learning." – Jean Watson

Is it possible that you can give yourself the same quality of care you give your patients?

What might that include?

...And You Might Try

We all tend to focus on what we did wrong. What about if at the end of the day you looked back and noted down everything you did well that day? You may want to start a "small victories this past week" journal. I find this especially helpful in times of high stress.

Chapter 11:
Riding the Sea Change

Rather, ten times, die in the surf, heralding the way to a new world, than stand idly on the shore.

– Florence Nightingale (2020)

Service and Survival

The call to service can provide an interesting ride. Sometimes it means to serve at one hospital for an entire career. For others it may entail travel nursing. Still others answer the call by working for the same doctor and building long-term relationships with the patients. Routine is comfortable, but sometimes life throws us a blindside hit. We have a choice as to how we respond.

It is how we respond to change that affects how we survive. Resilience, rebounding in the face of adversity, is the key. Finding the strength within can keep us going whether the adversity is personal or professional.

Viktor Frankl first wrote about choice as the ultimate freedom, based on his experience as a survivor at Auschwitz concentration camp (2006). Observation and personal experience led him to the realization that how we choose to respond is something that can never be stolen from us. "Everything can be taken from a man but one thing: the last of the human freedoms — to choose one's attitude in any given set of circumstances, to choose one's own way" (2006, p. 66).

Frankl's experience was based on his response to unimaginable conditions. In little ways, each of us is repeatedly faced with choice in daily life. Am I going to be mad at the person who cut me off as I drove to work? Am I going to carry that anger with me throughout the day? Or will I just blast it out at the first person who crosses me at work or at home? How we react is our choice.

My Story, Yet Again

In August 2019, I was on my way to a spiritual retreat in Italy. This trip was a dream come true. I'd left home that morning at 5:00 a.m., but my departure to Rome from JFK airport in New York had been repeatedly delayed. I dozed off around midnight. When I awoke, the plane was gone!

To make matters worse, even though I was physically there I was considered a no-show. My ticket could not be changed or refunded, and my return flight home from New

York was a week away. It was now 1:00 a.m., and everything was closed. I was on unknown turf, so the safest option seemed to be to sit in the empty terminal with other travelers. I am sure many of them had their own tales of travel misadventures. I waited for daylight; thinking of options fueled me.

I didn't want to just go home. It would have felt like defeat. I decided to make the best of it. Because it was cheaper than an extra ticket home, I rented a car and spent the week reconnecting with old friends along the East Coast. Each morning I said, "Okay, God. What's up today?" Every day was an adventure, as one spontaneous event led to another.

As I stood in the rental car parking lot, I released my attachment to my carefully planned week-long retreat in Italy. I let it go and trusted in God's presence in the outcome. I wasn't afraid. I wasn't anxious. I was curious how this would all unfold. I knew God was with me. I wasn't alone.

The first person who came to mind was an old friend with whom I was out of touch. I called, and she said she had been thinking of me as she faced unexpected surgery for a brain aneurism. She thought of calling me but fretted that I was too busy. And besides, she thought I still lived in New Orleans. I immediately headed south to her home outside of Baltimore to provide whatever support that I could.

A couple of days later, I drove back to New York City. The trip became a sentimental journey as I visited the places where my husband James and I lived when we were first married. I visited another home we shared in New Jersey. I stayed with my Mississippi-born niece who lives in Brooklyn and got to connect with her as an adult. In Manhattan, I was on my way to catch the "A" train to our old neighborhood when a call came from some pastor friends. They had seen me in the crowd at *The Today Show* and knew I was in town. With them, I ate seafood on the Long Island Sound and put my toes in the ocean. Another day, I toured the New York harbor with one of my New Orleans nurses who is now a traveling nurse.

It was a week of triumph, not defeat, because I allowed myself to be led by my Inner Teacher. Instead of focusing on the worst, I opened myself up to a different experience. I chose to make something better happen, and it did. And through an amazing series of events, my plane ticket was refunded. I didn't even lose my money for the retreat! The monastery agreed to hold my tuition for 2020.

Once again, I found that the universe will jump in to help, if we only get ourselves out of the way. I trusted that it would all work out, and it did, in a way that was so much better than I could ever have imagined. I am reminded of the old saying that there are three answers to prayer: "Yes. No. Not now, but later."

My trust that a good outcome can come from change was acquired through experience over a lifelong process of self-examination, faith, and optimism. This maturation process has not always been easy.

Facing the Tough Stuff

The single most radical change in my life happened as my husband James and I sat in the marriage counselor's office in October 1989. We counted ourselves among the lucky ones. James worked at Opryland Hotel in Nashville, Tennessee. One of the perks of his job was a free, on-site counseling service. James and I were there after a major shouting match in the backyard as I hung clothes out to dry. It was a week after our twelfth anniversary, and here we were at the counselor's office. We had a pleasant enough time talking to him, but a part of me felt like we were doing a beautiful job of pretending to be better than we were.

Then James did it. He changed the course of our life together. It was like he was standing on the high dive and he dove in. It took my breath away to watch. As we were closing down the meeting he said, "I think I've developed a drinking problem."

There was a moment when that statement just hung in the air. James named the proverbial elephant in the room. I, on the other hand, thought, "Oh, I'm so glad he remembered to

181

mention that!" (Did I mention that my first initial is D for Dorothy? It could also stand for Denial.)

The appointment was on Tuesday, and James went into treatment on Friday. It was so inconvenient. James was a bellman. He made $2.00 an hour plus tips. This was the good old days when in-patient treatment lasted a month. How could we live without his tips?

And I Thought the Problem Was Him

Even more personal was the question, "What about me?" It is one thing to expect James to change. As the process unfolded, a realization washed over me. I was going to have to change too.

I remember thinking, "I don't want to be left behind!" I was going to have to look at my own shadows of sexual abuse and food issues to figure out why I married an alcoholic. I hadn't grown up around alcohol. I just never thought drinking six beers a day could mean a person was an alcoholic, and I certainly didn't understand all the parts of our lives that our sicknesses affected.

There were a lot of obstacles, but somehow it all fell into place. It was as if James asked for help, and the angels rushed in to deposit him in the Rehab Unit of Baptist Hospital in Nashville, Tennessee. We celebrated our son's fourth birthday there.

Change happens, and we don't always have control over what comes our way. Some changes are small in the grand scheme of life, like my choosing to explore the Atlantic seaboard after missing my plane. Other changes can feel like life or death. James' diagnosis created a change that had repercussions in every facet of our life together.

Indeed, some necessary changes are profound and require a complete paradigm shift. In *The Spiritual Journey* (1990), Coombs and Nemeck state that there are three critical thresholds to be crossed as one continues to grow. The threshold is that part of the doorway that connects two rooms; meeting the challenge of change can be like crossing over to a new phase of life. Some are more important than others. These authors describe three that are considered critical elements of human development:

1. They are radical. James admitting his drinking problem was radical. He didn't weigh the repercussions. He didn't stop to wonder how I would react. He was fighting for his life, and we were welcomed to come along with him. To admit a problem like that creates change right down to the molecular level.

2. They are irreversible. Once he named the problem, there was no going back. As the old saying goes, "the cat was out of the bag," and no way it could go back in. His admission was like throwing a stone in a pond and watching the waves move out from the central point. The resulting changes

183

touched everyone in our family. Were we, as a family, willing to change too?

3. They are successive. One threshold builds on the previous one and opens the path to another. Generally, it is like a ladder that must be climbed one rung at a time. Consistency is hard, but it is essential for lasting change. That's one of the biggest challenges for all of us.

Accepting the Possibilities

Change can be inconvenient and sometimes scary, but there is one big question. Are you willing to change? Are you willing to try something new? It may be something as simple as taking a slightly longer but more scenic way home from work. Or it may be a big life change. Will you let it break you, or can you find the good in even the most difficult situations?

Some things are out of our control, like the plane that left without me or James's diagnosis of alcoholism. As bad as those events were when I was in the middle of them, I can look back and reflect on how they each became an avenue for change and growth in my life. I see clearly how God placed in our paths people who helped or opportunities to look at things in a different way. It is important to let the heart lead you and to step out in faith when opportunities inevitably arise. It is up to us to accept them or reject them.

Job or Profession?

The general conception is that a job is work for which we get paid. We show up, do the work, and get a check or an automatic deposit. The job may require training or special skills. Hopefully, it is something we enjoy, but there may be certain aspects of the job that do not appeal to us. We might like the folks we work with and find the outcome satisfying. But at the end of the day, the work ends when we go home.

How we feel about the work we do is important because it is a part of who we are. We all are called to meaningful work. Or as Frankl states,

"Everyone has his own specific vocation or mission in life; everyone must carry out a concrete assignment that demands fulfillment. Therein he cannot be replaced, nor can his life be repeated. Thus, everyone's task is unique as is his specific opportunity to implement it." (2006, p. 109)

A profession takes a job a step deeper because it is a commitment not only to a type of work, but to a way of life. Nursing on any level is not just a job, it is a profession. Becoming a part of a profession means that you have met all the standards of its governing body. You completed rigorous training, learned the language of your profession, passed your boards, and have been prepared to practice. That is the beginning, and there is more.

My profession is chaplaincy, which is under the umbrella of ministry. The call to serve is my guiding light. The call was first formally expressed in church ministry, but then it led me beyond the physical walls of the church to climb on oil rigs, to enter manufacturing plants, to offer support to families following Hurricane Katrina, and finally, to sit at the bedside of critically ill patients. Now, I hold the hands of families as they consider the incredibly selfless decision to give others the Gift of Life through organ donation with Kentucky Organ Donation Affiliates.

The type of work I do requires extensive training, patience, and personal commitment. When you buy a house or car and pledge to the bank that you will pay back the loan, that is one form of commitment. Personal commitment is making a pledge to yourself and to your world that this is a duty you are willing to give your life to.

When I first began my journey toward ordination as a minister, someone told me that it takes about ten years to fully "become" the profession. What they meant was that a profession is an all-encompassing lifestyle, and it takes a while to fully embrace the professional role you have or will become. At the time I first heard the statement, I found it irritating. After all, look at the training I had and the life experience I was bringing to my work! I see the truth in it now. Those first ten years were part of the preparation. They brought me to my chaplain residency and to my doctoral work with "my" nurses. We agreed to their anonymity, but their names are written on my heart.

The other big difference between a profession and a job, is the power that comes with the profession. Yes, nurses hold tremendous power. You may laugh and roll your eyes at that thought as you remember your last shift, but you are an essential and respected part of healthcare. In whatever you do – at bedside, in the doctor's office, in the emergency room, or in any phase of nursing – you hold power in other's lives. No matter what your personal beliefs may be, the nurse/patient relationship is sacred. You are the advocate and the voice for your patients in the most vulnerable moments of their lives. You may not feel powerful, but your healing presence certainly is.

From 2001 to 2018, the Gallup poll has undertaken gauging public perception of ethical behavior in twenty professions in the United States. The results? Nurses have consistently placed as number one – over doctors, pharmacists, teachers, and police officers. You are trusted, and you are entrusted with the care of others.

Much like a snake outgrows and sheds its skin, growing into your profession is a series of steps that goes far beyond acquiring skills. Technically, there will always be something new to learn, for as long as you want to keep working.

Learning is good even when it is not especially fun. Learning works the brain and keeps you sharp. Are there ways you can challenge yourself and keep from getting bored with your job?

Service and Survival II

Jobs may come, and jobs may go. But the essence of who you are is expressed in your profession. It is your foundation. It is essential that you protect that core part of you as you would protect a newborn child. That is where your Wisdom lies. If you minimize it or ignore it, then the part of you that sustains you will shrivel and give way to dreaded burnout.

In 2019, the World Health Organization included burnout as an occupational phenomenon in the 11th Revision of the International Classification of Diseases (ICD-11), describing it as follows:

"Burn-out is a syndrome conceptualized as resulting from chronic workplace stress that has not been successfully managed. It is characterized by three dimensions: feelings of energy depletion or exhaustion; increased mental distance from one's job, or feelings of negativism or cynicism related to one's job; and reduced professional efficacy."

The work you do is often physically and emotionally difficult. Is there someplace where you can go, either physically or mentally, where you feel restored? Maybe just a few minutes in the breakroom for a "time out" is all you need to face the next task at hand. Take that moment. Claim it for its value.

A ritual is a gesture that holds special meaning. Religions have rituals to mark changes in life, like marriage or death. Sometimes establishing a ritual for yourself can help you keep a clear mind. I shared with you my hand sanitizer ritual. Before I enter the room, I take a breath as I pump the dispenser. I breathe in to restore myself. I breathe out to clear myself from the previous patient or task. I am cleared for the next task at hand.

Mindfulness is simply being aware. Remembering to be aware is sometimes difficult, especially when you are busy in the middle of the day. What simple action could you use to ground yourself intermittently throughout the day?

Deep Listening Leads to Deep Connection

And of course, listening is essential to the practice of your craft. Remember, hearing engages the mind. Listening engages the heart. Your attention shows your intention to listen, and that opens the door to deeper connection, not only with the patient but also with their families, the staff you work with, and those you have at home.

One study nurse said that through her intentional listening, she was able to help other members of the team. A young male patient had a tracheostomy "and people were getting frustrated trying to talk to him. It took so long for him to write out everything." The nurse said that she felt that she was able to slow herself down to better communicate with him, and she encouraged others to slow their pace too. "Being patient provided a better atmosphere for communication, and as I was telling [the nurses], we were listening in more ways than just words." She indicated that use of the model helped her provide better leadership in a difficult situation (Participant #6).

Listening is a skill taught in the nursing curriculum, and you most likely do it consistently well. Deep listening is another skill that can be learned, and the results benefit both you and your patients. One of the study nurses shared trying to use the model at home as she spoke with her husband and adult daughter. She laughed and said her husband was definitely *not* using the Quaker Listening Method! She confided, "I think before I learned this, I wouldn't have been able to put my finger on why exactly this conversation was going down the tubes... It is very concrete and practical. That's what I really liked about this model" (Participant #10).

In the Garden

Remember the image of the two gardens? The neat and orderly vegetable garden, like Mr. McGregor's garden in *The Tale of Peter Rabbit*, reflects the organized left brain that takes information and categorizes it within an established system. The left brain is the seat of the personality or the "I," which is the way we present ourselves to the world.

The other verdant, thick, and richly colorful messy garden is more like the jungle in Maurice Sendak's *Where the Wild Things Are*. That garden reflects our immediate responses to stimuli. The images go through that ever-swinging two-way gate, to the left brain which categorizes them. The jungle garden represents the "We," that collective mind we share. Connecting with that right side of the brain is where the connection to the Soul or Inner Teacher lies.

Habit may take us to the comfortable left side of the brain, where the personality holds the reins and where our logical mind runs the show. However, if we can catch ourselves and pause before heading to the left brain, there is an invitation to respond and not just react. That invitation can easily be overlooked. It is the invitation from that rich and unruly part of the brain to connect, human-to-human, with the patient on a deeper level.

Remember this. A question is an invitation. If a patient asks a question, they are inviting you to engage and connect.

Perhaps that connection, that reminder of our shared humanity, will be your respite from an overwhelming day.

Your response is a choice. Will you choose to scratch the surface or to dig a little bit deeper? That is my invitation to you.

Now... How did you come to be a nurse?

About the Author

Rev. Dr. Clare Biedenharn is a board certified chaplain with over two decades of chaplaincy experience, both in industry and critical care. She was first an industrial chaplain, wearing a hard hat and climbing on oil rigs. From there she transitioned to the bedside in a hospital critical care setting. Now her focus is on supporting families as they face end-of-life care decisions about organ donation.

Through her years of hands-on experience, Clare came to embrace the belief that intentional listening is an essential element of care. That idea formed the foundation of her study with critical care nurses.

"Life-long learner" is a moniker Clare is proud to claim. Her listening study was not only a labor of love, it fulfilled requirements for the Doctor of Ministry in Spiritual Direction (D.Min.) degree from Garrett Theological Seminary in Evanston, Illinois, from which she also holds a M.A. in Spiritual Formation. In addition, she holds an Ed.S. in Adult Learning from the University of Southern Mississippi, with a focus on spirituality in the hospital setting. She is also an ordained minister in the United Methodist Church and served the local church for ten years before entering full-time chaplaincy.

Clare is Board Certified through the Association of Professional Chaplains and holds a Palliative Care Chaplaincy Specialty certificate from California State University Institute for Palliative Care.

Clare called on every skill at her disposal as she cared for her husband James. He succumbed to a rare thymic cancer in 2018 after a four-year battle. James encouraged her to return to her listening project after his death, and so she has.

She has two adult sons, Jay and Robert, who were each wise enough to marry smart and loving women. Three wonderful grandchildren bless her life.

Further information on Clare's listening project is available at YourListeningPartner.com.

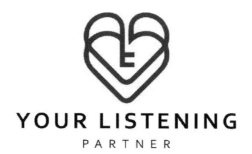

YOUR LISTENING
PARTNER

A Special Thank You Gift

From Dr. Clare Biedenharn

Now that you've got your copy of Heart to Heart: Spiritual Care Through Deep Listening, you've begun a journey toward deeper connection to both your personal and professional life. This intentional listening model has worked for others for over 400 years and it can work for you.

Deep listening leads to deep connection. Deep connection leads to transformation. As you use the tools in this book and reconnect with who you are as a healer, you might remember that tug on your heart that led you to commit your life to a special kind of service.

It all begins with an open, honest question.

You have many tools in your toolbox already. Let me offer you another.

We all need a little help now and then. So, I've created a special downloadable pocket card that you can carry with you. Included on it are hints to help you stay grounded throughout the day along with suggestions for questions to get you started.

You are seasoned professionals and know that listening is an essential part of nursing. This book provides a method of listening as well as specifics for providing the quality of spiritual care you may not have considered possible.

While this pocket card is offered for sale, as a special thank you please can claim it for free here:

http://yourlisteningpartner.com

The sooner you know process, the better your chances for experiencing the transformation that can come from deep connection with your patient and with your life.

I'm in your corner. Let me know if I can help further.

Wishing you the very best as you begin your journey.

Best,

Dr. Clare

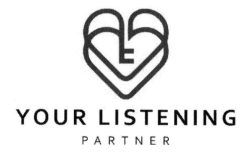

YOUR LISTENING
PARTNER

References

Active listening. U.S. Department of State. (2009). Retrieved 17 March 2013, from https://2009-2017.state.gov/m/a/os/65759.htm.

Anandarajah, G., & Hight, E. (2001). Spirituality and medical practice: using the HOPE questions as a practical tool for spiritual assessment. *American Family Physician*, *63*(1), 81-89.

Bevis, E., & Watson, J. (2000). *Toward a caring curriculum.* Jones and Bartlett Learning.

Biedenharn, D. (2014). A study of critical care nurses' listening behavior through the application of the Quaker listening model (D.Min.). Garrett Theological Seminary.

Bolte-Taylor, J. (2008). *My stroke of insight.* TED. Retrieved 17 February 2018, from https://www.ted.com/talks/jill_bolte_taylor_my_stroke_of_insight.

Bolte-Taylor, J. (2009). *My stroke of insight.* Plume.

Bostridge, M. (2008). *Florence Nightingale: The making of an Icon.* Farrar, Straus and Giroux.

Burn-out an "occupational phenomenon": International classification of diseases. World Health Organization.

(2019). Retrieved 13 December 2019, from
https://www.who.int/mental_health/evidence/burn-out/en/.

Cocker, F., & Joss, N. (2016). Compassion fatigue among
healthcare, emergency and community service workers: A
systematic review. *International Journal of
Environmental Research and Public Health, 13*(6), 618.
https://doi.org/10.3390/ijerph13060618

Coombs, M., & Nemeck, OMI, F. (1990). *The spiritual
journey*. Liturgical Press.

Crick, R., & Miller, B. (2011). Outside the gates: Theology,
history and practice of chaplain ministries. HigherLife
Publishing.

Dossey, B. (2001). *Florence Nightingale lecture by Barbara
Dossey*. Dosseydossey.com. Retrieved 17 November 2019,
from
http://www.dosseydossey.com/barbara/floranceLecture.ht
ml.

FAQs. Friends General Conference. (2018). Retrieved 17
October 2018, from
https://www.fgcquaker.org/discover/faqs-about-quakers.

Frankl, V. (2006). *Man's search for meaning*. Beacon Press.

Freire, P. (1968). *Pedagogy of the oppressed*. Continuum.

Gallup, I. (2018). *Nurses again outpace other professions for
honesty, ethics*. Gallup.com. Retrieved 17 November 2019,

from https://news.gallup.com/poll/245597/nurses-again-outpace-professions-honesty-ethics.aspx.

Graham, E., Walton, H., Ward, F., & Stuerzenhofecker, K. (2005). *Theological reflections: Methods*. SCM Press.

Hamm, T. (2003). *The Quakers in America*. Columbia University Press.

Hodge, D. (2006). A template for spiritual assessment: A review of the JCAHO requirements and guidelines for implementation. *Social Work*, *51*(4), 317-326. https://doi.org/10.1093/sw/51.4.317

Jenkins, M., Wikoff, K., Amankwaa, L., & Trent, B. (2009). Nursing the spirit. *Nursing Management (Springhouse)*, *40*(8), 29-36. https://doi.org/10.1097/01.numa.0000359206.44705.b6

Johnson, M. (2018). *Nurse Tamara Ferguson's harrowing story of surviving the California wildfire*. GodUpdates. Retrieved 18 December 2019, from https://www.godupdates.com/california-nurse-tamara-ferguson-wildfire-heroic-story/.

Lewis, D. (2008). *The Joint Commission and spiritual care | Spiritual Directors International*. Sdiworld.org. Retrieved 23 December 2019, from https://www.sdiworld.org/blog/joint-commission-and-spiritual-care.

Maruca, S. (2020). *Walking together in faith*. Donghanh-
online.blogspot.com. Retrieved 17 February 2020, from
http://donghanh-online.blogspot.com/2009/10/walking-
together-in-faith.html.

McDonald, L. (2010). *Florence Nightingale at first hand*.
Continuum International Pub.

Moore, T. (1992). Care of the Soul: A Guide for Cultivating
Depth and Sacredness. HarperCollins.

Nightingale, F. (1973). *A 'note' of interrogation*. Maths-
people.anu.edu.au. Retrieved 20 December 2019, from
https://maths-people.anu.edu.au/~johnm/misc/FN/frasers-
may73.pdf.

Nightingale, F. (2001). *Notes on nursing: What it is and what
it is not*. University of Michigan Library.

Nightingale, F. (2015). *Florence Nightingale to her nurses*.
Echo Library.

Nightingale, F. (2019). *A conversation with Florence
Nightingale*. Aacn.org. Retrieved 18 April 2019, from
https://www.aacn.org/nursing-excellence/nurse-stories/a-
conversation-with-florence-nightingale.

Nightingale, F. (2020). *Our 20 favorite Florence Nightingale
quotes*. Electronic Medical Certification. Retrieved 17
December 2019, from https://emedcert.com/blog/20-
favorite-florence-nightingale-quotes.

Nursing Management. (2009), *30*(11), 29-36.
https://doi.org/10.1097/01.NUMA.0000359206.44705.b6

Oxford Essential Quotations. (2016).
https://doi.org/10.1093/acref/9780191826719.001.0001

Palmer, P. (2007). The courage to teach: Exploring the inner
landscape of a teacher's life. Jossey-Bass.

Palmer, P. (2009). *A hidden wholeness*. Jossey-Bass/Wiley.

Palmer, P. (2013). *What is an undivided life?* Center for
Courage & Renewal. Retrieved 10 December 2013, from
http://www.couragerenewal.org/stories/what-is-a-divided-
life/.

Pigott, J., Hargreaves, J., & Power, J. (2016). *Liminal
hospital spaces: Corridors to well-being?* The Third
International Conference Exploring Multi-Dimensions of
Well-Being. Retrieved 19 December 2019, from
http://eprints.hud.ac.uk/id/eprint/29567/1/57%20Pigott%2
0J%20%20FULL%20PAPER%20Liminal%20Hospital%20
Spaces%20%20Corridors%20to%20Well-Being_.pdf.

Potter, B. (2008). *Peter Rabbit*. Frederick Warne.

Puchalski, C., & Ferrell, B. (2010). *Making health care whole:
Integrating spirituality into health care*. Templeton Press.

RCN Spirituality Survey 2010. Royal Academy of Nursing.
(2011). Retrieved 17 October 2019, from

https://www.rcn.org.uk/professional-development/publications/pub-003861.

Sendak, M. (1988). *Where the wild things are.* Harper & Row.

Smith-Stoner, M. (2011). *Teaching patient-centered care during the silver hour.* Medscape. Retrieved 17 February 2020, from http://www.medscape.com/viewarticle/751640_7.

Stairs, J. (2001). *Listening for the soul.* Fortress Press.

The Social Justice Testimony | Quaker Information Center. Quakerinfo.org. (2020). Retrieved 24 February 2020, from https://quakerinfo.org/quakerism/social-justice.

Underwood, L. (2003). *Multidimensional measurement of religious spirituality for use in health research.* Fetzer.org. Retrieved 17 February 2013, from https://fetzer.org/sites/default/files/resources/attachment/%5Bcurrent-date%3Atiny%5D/Multidimensional_Measurement_of_Religiousness_Spirituality.pdf.

Valizadeh, L., Jasemi, M., Zamanzadeh, V., & Keogh, B. (2017). A Concept Analysis of Holistic Care by Hybrid Model. *Indian Journal of Palliative Care, 23*(1), 71. https://doi.org/10.4103/0973-1075.197960

Vance, R. (2020). *Caring and the professional practice of nursing.* rn-journal.com. Retrieved 23 March 2013, from https://rn-journal.com/journal-of-nursing/caring-and-the-professional-practice-of- nursing.

Vedantam, S. (2019). *In the heat of the moment: How intense emotions transforms us.* Hidden Brain [Podcast]. Retrieved 2 December 2019, from http://https:www.npr.org/transcripts/783495595.

Walking together in faith. Donghanh-online.blogspot.com. (2020). Retrieved 17 December 2019, from http://donghanh-online.blogspot.com/2009/10/walking-together-in-faith.html.

Watson, J. (2010). *Core concepts.* Watson Caring Science. Retrieved 1 February 2014, from https://www.watsoncaringscience.org/files/PDF/watsons-theory-of-human-caring-core-concepts-and-evolution-to-caritas-processes-handout.pdf.

Watson, J. (2010). *Nursing: Philosophy and science of caring.* University Press of Colorado.

Watson, J. (2020). *Assumptions.* Jean Watson: Caring Science. Retrieved 17 February 2014, from https://jeanwatsoncaringscience.weebly.com/assumptions.html.

Wesley, J. (2010). *Primitive physick* (14th ed.). Gale Ecco, Print Editions.

Wesley, J. *The Wesley Center Online: Sermon 98 - On visiting the sick.* Wesley.nnu.edu. (2020). Retrieved 17 February

2020, from http://wesley.nnu.edu/john-wesley/the-sermons-of-john-wesley-1872-edition/sermon-98-on-visiting-the-sick/.

Index

Abraham, biblical, 41
Adventist Feather Hospital, 34
Affordable Care Act, 146
agape, 166
Anandarajah, Gowri, 60
Ark of the Covenant, 80
assessment
    of nurse by patient, 94
    patient, 61, 126, 130, 147, 163
    spiritual, 39, 48, 57, 58, 61, 62
    spiritual, with FICA acronym, 59
    spiritual, with HOPE acronym, 59
    visual, 69
Association of Professional
    Chaplains, 17, 40, 218
attention, conscious use of, 69, 99,
    131, 135, 138, 146, 152, 185, 193,
    212
aura, 95
Banjo, 107, 108
Bevis, Em Olivia, 61, 87, 168
bias
    as a filter, 90, 111, 130
    professional, 50, 51
Biedenharn, Clare, 9, 10, 13, 217,
    221
Biedenharn, James, ii, 202, 203, 204,
    205, 206, 207, 218
Biedenharn, Jay, ii, 218
Biedenharn, Robert, ii, iii, 116, 218
Bihm, Barbara, iv
Block, Donna, iv
Board Certified Chaplain, 13, 17, 40
body
    language, nonverbal communication
        through, 138, 155

    physical response to stimulus, 169,
        170
Bolte-Taylor, Jill, 100, 101, 102, 157,
    158, 159, 166, 169, 179
brain
    connection between hemispheres, 158
    corpus callosum, 158, 160, 163
    left hemisphere, 159, 160, 163, 164,
        214, 215
    right hemisphere, 158, 159, 160, 163
Buddhism, 63, 76
burnout, 105, 211
burnout, 106
burnout, 211
burnout, 211
California State University Institute
    for Palliative Care, 218
call to service, 19, 24, 34, 36, 37, 38,
    42, 98, 106, 110, 166, 199, 208
Caring Moment, 168
chaplaincy, 9, 10, 52, 73, 74, 105, 156,
    182, 208, 217, 218
    as practical theology, 74
    critical care, i, 101, 104, 217
    critical care, 19
    end of life care, 217
    hospital, 16, 39, 40, 68, 74
    industrial, 16, 17, 104, 118, 217
    industry, 217
    military, 16
Chicago, Illinois, 37
Christianity, 43, 63, 76, 109
    Methodism, 114
Clearness Committee, 24, 25, 29,
    121, 126, 174, 175, 176, 177, 178,
    180, 181, 186
    Role of, 176
    Seeker, role of, 175, 176, 177

205

Made in the USA
Columbia, SC
02 June 2020